Professor Kevin Gournay CBE is a registered psychologist, chartered scientist and a registered nurse who is an emeritus professor at the Institute of Psychiatry, King's College, London. Over more than 35 years, he has had extensive clinical experience in the treatment of adult and child victims of post-traumatic stress. He has been responsible for the assessment and treatment of people who have been through a range of traumatic events. These include the Moorgate tube accident (1975), the King's Cross fire (1987), the sinking of the *Herald of Free Enterprise* ferry (1987), the Paddington and Potters Bar rail crashes (1995 and 2002), and the terrorist bombings of 2005. He has also treated and assessed people involved in various domestic, industrial and road traffic accidents and other trauma, including war- and crime-related events and medical negligence.

Overcoming Common Problems Series

Selected titles

A full list of titles is available from Sheldon Press,
36 Causton Street, London SW1P 4ST and on our website at
www.sheldonpress.co.uk

Breast Cancer: Your treatment choices
Dr Terry Priestman

Chronic Fatigue Syndrome: What you need to know about CFS/ME
Dr Megan A. Arroll

Cider Vinegar
Margaret Hills

Coping Successfully with Chronic Illness: Your healing plan
Neville Shone

Coping Successfully with Hiatus Hernia
Dr Tom Smith

Coping with Difficult Families
Dr Jane McGregor and Tim McGregor

Coping with Epilepsy
Dr Pamela Crawford and Fiona Marshall

Coping with Guilt
Dr Windy Dryden

Coping with Liver Disease
Mark Greener

Coping with Memory Problems
Dr Sallie Baxendale

Coping with Obsessive Compulsive Disorder
Professor Kevin Gournay, Rachel Piper and Professor Paul Rogers

Coping with the Psychological Effects of Illness
Dr Fran Smith, Dr Carina Eriksen and Professor Robert Bor

Coping with Schizophrenia
Professor Kevin Gournay and Debbie Robson

Coping with Thyroid Disease
Mark Greener

Depressive Illness: The curse of the strong
Dr Tim Cantopher

The Empathy Trap: Understanding antisocial personalities
Dr Jane McGregor and Tim McGregor

Epilepsy: Complementary and alternative treatments
Dr Sallie Baxendale

The Fibromyalgia Healing Diet
Christine Craggs-Hinton

Fibromyalgia: Your treatment guide
Christine Craggs-Hinton

Hay Fever: How to beat it
Dr Paul Carson

Helping Elderly Relatives
Jill Eckersley

The Holistic Health Handbook
Mark Greener

How to Eat Well When You Have Cancer
Jane Freeman

How to Stop Worrying
Dr Frank Tallis

Invisible Illness: Coping with misunderstood conditions
Dr Megan A. Arroll and Professor Christine P. Dancey

Living with Complicated Grief
Professor Craig A. White

Living with Fibromyalgia
Christine Craggs-Hinton

Living with Hearing Loss
Dr Don McFerran, Lucy Handscomb and Dr Cherilee Rutherford

Living with IBS
Nuno Ferreira and David T. Gillanders

Overcoming Fear: With mindfulness
Deborah Ward

Overcoming Stress
Professor Robert Bor, Dr Carina Eriksen and Dr Sara Chaudry

Overcoming Worry and Anxiety
Dr Jerry Kennard

Physical Intelligence: How to take charge of your weight
Dr Tom Smith

The Self-Esteem Journal
Alison Waines

The Stroke Survival Guide
Mark Greener

Ten Steps to Positive Living
Dr Windy Dryden

Treating Arthritis: The drug-free way
Margaret Hills and Christine Horner

Treating Arthritis: The supplements guide
Julia Davies

Understanding Yourself and Others: Practical ideas from the world of coaching
Bob Thomson

When Someone You Love Has Depression: A handbook for family and friends
Barbara Baker

Overcoming Common Problems

Post-Traumatic Stress Disorder
Recovery after accident and disaster

PROFESSOR KEVIN GOURNAY

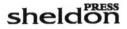

First published in Great Britain in 2015

Sheldon Press
36 Causton Street
London SW1P 4ST
www.sheldonpress.co.uk

British Library Cataloguing-in-Publication Data
A catalogue record for this book is available from the British Library

ISBN 978–1–84709–320–2
eBook ISBN 978–1–84709–321–9

Typeset by Fakenham Prepress Solutions, Fakenham, Norfolk NR21 8NN
First printed in Great Britain by Ashford Colour Press.
Subsequently digitally reprinted in Great Britain

eBook by Fakenham Prepress Solutions, Fakenham, Norfolk NR21 8NN

Produced on paper from sustainable forests

For my dad Joe (1917–2010),
an unsung hero – of the Second World War and other things,
but most of all a hero to his children,
Kevin, Bernard (1948–2013) and Imelda

Contents

Acknowledgements

My professional life, spanning more than four decades, has been blessed by contact with so many wonderful people – professionals, clinicians and academics – who have taught me so much, not just about the subject of this book but about psychiatry and psychology in general. I was also privileged to have spent a great deal of my working life at what is arguably the best psychiatric research institution in the world, the Institute of Psychiatry at the Maudsley Hospital, at King's College, London. Therefore there are simply too many individuals to thank and name, and if I attempted to do so I am sure I would leave someone out. However, I wish to mention some people who have provided me with particular inspiration, encouragement and education.

First and foremost I thank Isaac Marks, now an Emeritus Professor who, through the groundbreaking training programme in Behavioural Psychotherapy – now rebranded as cognitive behavioural therapy (CBT) – gave me the skills and knowledge that I have used to pursue my career, not only as a clinician but also as a researcher, teacher and policy adviser. Isaac inculcated in me the recognition that one needs to be aware of the background evidence for any treatment approach. He also taught me the value of dealing with each individual in a pragmatic way and to use hunches and intuition when designing treatment.

Professor Kevin Howells supervised my own MPhil and PhD, which had a primary focus on the evaluation of exposure therapy – one of the central interventions for post-traumatic stress disorder (PTSD). As with so many things, it is now, more than 30 years on, that I recognize the way his quiet encouragement provided me with the opportunity to begin to develop my skills as a researcher. I will be forever grateful to him for his supervision of not one but two theses.

Later on in my development I was fortunate to have Professor Sir David Goldberg as my boss at the Institute of Psychiatry – a role taken over by Professor Graham Thornicroft in the second part of my professorial tenure. Sir David enthused me not only through his massive intellect and reservoir of knowledge but by his great sense of humour and, at times, his gross political incorrectness! David is certainly one of those individuals who can make one think of the world in a different way. Following David's retirement, Graham Thornicroft also served as a source of inspiration. Of very different character from David, Graham's careful, systematic approach to psychiatric research also served to make me see things differently.

I also want to mention my current sources of stimulation and inspiration. Two of my clinical colleagues, Dr David Veale and Dr Mike Beary (both psychiatrists), have also, in their own ways, helped me along my pathway of learning. For their contributions I am most grateful. I assisted David Veale some 20 or more years ago in the development of a treatment model for body dysmorphic disorder. This collaboration made me begin to think about the value of cognitive models for treatment, but also to wonder about genetic and environmental contributions to thinking processes – a phenomenon now of great importance in our understanding of psychiatric illness. Mike Beary provides me with wise counsel in my work as a clinician; he is first and foremost a kind, caring physician who has reinforced in me the need to see the physical as well as the psychological in my patients.

Over the past 20 years I have enjoyed the wide-ranging collaboration and friendship of Professor Maree Teesson and her husband Dr Andrew Baillee, in Sydney, Australia. Currently I work with both Maree and Andrew on a large portfolio of projects concerning the comorbidity of mental illness and drug and alcohol use. The projects, which include studies of PTSD in this population, have provided me with more ways of thinking. Maree and Andrew deserve particular thanks for different things. Maree, a true leader in her research and the policy field, has shown me how to think about what comes next in our quest for knowledge; she has also been one of the most vocal of advocates for increasing consumer involvement. Andrew, an outstanding polymath of a man, has rekindled my desire to call out – in many areas of psychiatry and particularly psychology – 'The Emperor has no clothes!' On a lighter note, both have made me feel – over the course of 22 visits – an honorary Australian.

I must also provide a different acknowledgement to, probably, a more important group of people. These are the hundreds of patients I have met, victims of traumatic stress – collectively similar but so very different and unique in their presentation. They have been my primary source of motivation in writing this book, which I hope will serve others in their quest for recovery.

My commissioning editor at Sheldon Press, Fiona Marshall, has been a pleasure to work with. She has been patient with the delays in delivery of manuscripts, not just of this book but the three previous ones I have written for Sheldon. Such delays are inevitable when combining clinical work with other endeavours.

None of these books would have been possible without the input of Kate, my much trusted and excellent secretary, who corrects my grammatical errors without complaint. To you, Kate, I owe much. Like my family, you have provided invaluable support. My sincere thanks also to Neil Whyte for his painstaking work in copy editing my manuscript on behalf of Sheldon Press. His input has been invaluable.

Finally, I must mention two central sources of inspiration for this book.

First, in work for the World Health Organization I visited Palestine and had the opportunity of meeting those touched – indeed traumatized – by the tragic events of the past few years. These encounters mirrored the accounts provided by two Jewish patients who had lost family members in bombings in Israel. Both experiences served to remind me that the innocent are the main victims of war and that war, no matter how righteous the cause, results in so much suffering.

Finally, my own father Joe (Joseph Louis), to whom this book is dedicated, has been in my mind throughout my writing. Joe spent much of his childhood caring for his mother, who was paralysed following surgery to remove a brain tumour. Before the Second World War, he went to a military college in France and subsequently enlisted in the Queen's Own Royal West Kent Regiment. He had met my mother, Eileen, and they became engaged. The Royal West Kents went to France as part of the British Expeditionary Force, and served as a rearguard for the troops evacuated from Dunkirk. Most of Joe's battalion were killed – 920 out of 1,000 men. My father was wounded by machine-gun fire; his life was saved by his backpack, which took a number of bullets. Nevertheless he was badly wounded and, after five days trying to escape, was eventually captured. Subsequently Joe spent two years in hospital and then two further years in a prisoner-of-war camp. During much of this time Joe was posted as 'Missing presumed dead'. Eventually, in 1944, Joe was repatriated by the Red Cross in an emaciated state. His homecoming, however, was joyous. He recalled being treated with great kindness by both German surgeons and soldiers during his time in hospital, and remembered how, while in the POW camp, as the war went on, his guards also suffered hunger. This, in a way, epitomized Joe's character: he saw the good in everyone and was always willing to see both sides of an argument. In retrospect it seems clear that his wartime experiences led him to remain a generally anxious individual, with a sense of vulnerability that became pronounced after my mother's death. At the same time he was blessed with a great sense of humour, a strong religious faith and the strongest of work ethics, which in turn provided benefit to his much loved family. Joe probably didn't qualify for the diagnosis of PTSD. However, as for millions of young men, war traumatized him.

A note of caution

While this book is intended to assist with coping with and recovery from trauma (with or without professional help), I realize that those with PTSD may well find the reading of some parts of this book difficult and, at times, possibly distressing. I know from my own experience that hearing the stories of others is, at once, distressing but also of comfort in knowing that one is not alone. Some parts of this book deal with particular signs and symptoms, and reading about these may set off thoughts and feelings that cause distress, discomfort, anxiety or other emotions. Although I hope that none of the above reactions occurs, I know that overcoming PTSD is often a painful process.

Although some people prefer to read a book from cover to cover or in large chunks, you might want to limit yourself to reading short sections at a time and then putting the book down and going on to other more pleasurable distractions. This is also a book that one can dip into, so when you look at the Contents or the Index, you might find a section that particularly applies to you – for example, coping with a particular feeling. By all means dip in and out but try, over time, to finish the entire book. Some of you may also find it helpful to make notes as you go along.

A final note of caution: should reading this book produce any overwhelming distress that does not readily subside once you have put down the book, you should, before continuing, discuss your reactions with your GP or, if you are undergoing treatment, with your therapist.

Introduction

Why yet another book on this subject?

The literature contains many sources of information and advice; nevertheless I feel that this is a book well worth writing for a number of reasons.

First, there is always a general need to update knowledge. In this respect, post-traumatic stress disorder is a condition for which treatments have developed apace in the past two decades. Thus there is a need for professionals and the general public alike to know about these developments.

My second reason for writing this book is to provide an account, from the perspective of a clinician, of the wide range of presentations coming under the umbrella of this diagnostic label. Since the 1970s I have encountered PTSD in hundreds of people, all with a unique presentation. It is worth emphasizing here that while diagnostic labels can be extremely helpful, sometimes they mask the individual perspective: no person presenting with this condition is the same – each has a unique experience and expresses distress in his or her own particular fashion.

Similarly, while there are guidelines for treatment and one can make generalized predictions about the outcome of treatment endeavours, there is no blueprint that can be applied to individual cases. One matter I wish to convey in this book is that, in my experience, there is often no correlation between the severity of a traumatic event and the consequences for an individual. Thus sometimes an accident that could be deemed trivial may have disastrous and lifelong consequences in respect of the PTSD suffered. On the other hand I have encountered individuals involved in the most horrific events who have emerged with either a very mild and transient form of PTSD or indeed no PTSD at all. So through the pages of this book I wish to convey what is sometimes very poorly described, particularly in the professional literature; that is, the need not only to address the general evidence that is available but also to pay heed to individuals and their particular circumstances. I will therefore use a number of case histories to illustrate how PTSD can present and how treatment may work.

My final reason for wishing to see this book in print has been formed by my experience of treating patients and recognizing their need to be provided with both information and advice, within one single publication. Until now I have needed to advise patients to read not one but several books and go to various websites to obtain the information and advice they need. My aspiration for this book is to put everything the individual needs to assist recovery together, under a single cover.

The case histories within this book

Throughout this book I have included case histories to illustrate a number of important points. All the descriptions come from my own clinical experience, gathered over more than three decades. However, I have protected the anonymity of particular patients not only by of course changing names but also by a process of interchanging parts of the history (that is, events and signs and symptoms). However, everything set out in the histories is true.

The word 'patient'

Throughout this book I use the word 'patient' rather than 'client' or indeed any of the other words or terms, such as 'consumer' or 'service user'. My work is within a hospital setting where 'patient' is the word used to designate those receiving treatment. In addition, research shows that the majority of people in receipt of such treatment prefer this word to describe them.

Part 1
ABOUT POST-TRAUMATIC STRESS DISORDER

1

The history and nature of PTSD

The history of the term post-traumatic stress disorder

Post-traumatic stress disorder (PTSD) is a relatively new term, introduced in 1980 by the American Psychiatric Association when it added this diagnostic category to the third edition of its *Diagnostic and Statistical Manual of Mental Disorders (DSM-III)*. Indeed the World Health Organization only began using the term in 1992. Nevertheless the phenomena coming under the diagnostic label of PTSD are by no means new. I recently found a very interesting reference to PTSD in an article by Steve Bentley (2005) reprinted in *The VVA Veteran*, the magazine of the Vietnam Veterans of America. This referred to the Greek historian Herodotus' writing of the battle of Marathon in 490 BC and describing an Athenian warrior becoming permanently blind when the soldier standing next to him was killed – the blinded soldier was 'wounded in no part of his body'. Bentley's article described PTSD over the centuries, up to the wars in Korea and Vietnam.

In the last century, Siegfried Sassoon and Wilfred Owen became famous for their poems describing the horrors of trench warfare. Sassoon and Owen met each other at Craiglockhart War Hospital near Edinburgh, where Sassoon took Owen under his wing. Both were deeply affected by their experiences of war yet both insisted on returning to the front. Owen died in action at the age of 25, just a week before the Armistice. For those interested in these poets I can strongly recommend the first part of Pat Barker's *Regeneration* trilogy, which gives a fictionalized account of the meeting of Sassoon and Owen (see the Further reading section at the end of this book).

It was recently pointed out to me that R. J. Daly described in an article clearly how, in the writings of the seventeenth-century British diarist Samuel Pepys, it is quite plain to see that he suffered from what we probably now recognize as PTSD following the Great Fire of London in 1666. It is evident from examination of Pepys' diary that it significantly affected him for some time. Pepys' first entry about the fire, as Daly's article tells us, was:

> 'Most horrid, malicious, blood fire ... So great was our fear ... It was enough to put us out of our wits.' He reported one week after the fire: 'Both sleeping and waking, and such fear of fire in my heart, that I took little rest.' While two weeks after the fire he wrote: 'Much terrified in the nights nowadays, with dreams of fire and falling down of houses.' Finally, six months after the fire, after noticing another chimney fire across London, he reported: 'put me into much fear and trouble ... still having night terrors'.

> (Daly 1983)

Over the years, what we now know as PTSD has been called by a number of terms, including war neurosis, shell shock and nervous shock. Indeed nervous shock is a term that has a specific legal meaning – a matter we will refer to later. PTSD is of course not limited to soldiers, and you will see in subsequent chapters that its causes, in respect of the specific traumatic stressors, are to be found in a wide range of events. The collective term PTSD describes a collection of signs and symptoms common to all those so afflicted. As we will see in some of the case histories, there are similarities between individuals in respect of the signs and symptoms experienced by people with PTSD, regardless of the event that caused it. Having said that, as I have noted above, each individual presents in a particular way – some symptoms, prominent in certain people, are not so troublesome in others.

As with many psychiatric terms, PTSD has been the subject of some misunderstanding, partly because of the way the meaning of particular words can change over time. 'Trauma' is now a very commonly used word associated with a variety of life events. Not to diminish the significance of these events in any way, trauma has unfortunately become associated with events such as examinations at school, finding that one has not been awarded a pay rise or even 'traumas' associated with positive events, such as choosing a wedding dress! Perhaps the best way to understand the difference between the trauma in PTSD and these everyday 'traumas' is to go back to some of the original definitions used in DSM III, which was mentioned above. In these definitions the event leading to PTSD was defined as something that was outside of the range of usual human experience and was an event that caused actual or threatened death, serious injury or threat to the physical integrity of self or others, and that the person who developed PTSD experienced, witnessed or was confronted with such an event. Having said all that, as we will see later on, the majority of us will experience such events over the course of a lifetime, although only a relatively small number will go on to develop PTSD. Any observer of psychiatry will note that psychiatric definitions not only change over time but are often the source of controversy. Asking a range of professionals with experience in cases of PTSD, from family doctors to solicitors and judges, will elicit a wide variety of opinions about the definitions. As we will also show in Chapter 4 on treatment, there is no 'right way' to treat PTSD; there are a number of approaches that are shown to have some effectiveness, but not everyone who is treated with 'effective treatment' recovers. Indeed it has been my experience that, for many, the main variables in the healing process can be found outside of psychiatry: in prayer within a particular religious belief, in the support found in others and, of course, in time itself. As we will discuss in subsequent chapters, some individuals – even those with severe levels of PTSD – can recover with the passage of time and without any particular professional intervention.

'Traumatic' – developing an understanding of the word in the context of PTSD

As I have noted above, trauma is a widely used word with different meanings for different people. Perhaps the best way to understand it in the context of the term 'post-traumatic stress disorder' is to turn to the latest definition of the American Psychiatric Association, in their *Diagnostic and Statistical Manual of Mental Disorders*, Fifth Edition, commonly known as *DSM-5*. This definition is now used universally by professionals, in both research and clinical practice. Although the World Health Organization also has a similar definition, the American Psychiatric Association's manual has a number of very helpful descriptions of PTSD and all its components. *DSM-5* states that the trigger for PTSD is exposure to actual or threatened death, serious injury or sexual violation. One of the key words here is 'threatened'. Thus the person may perceive the threat of death or serious injury, although from the outside such threats may be minimal. We shall take Paul's case as an example:

The case of Paul

As he had arrived home early from work, Paul picked up his seven-year-old daughter from school. It was a great pleasure to him to be able to meet his daughter Abigail at the end of the school day rather than seeing her when he usually arrived home tired from a day at work and stressful commuting. While he was waiting in the car, Paul mused over the joy that his daughter had brought to him and his wife since her birth. He made her safe and secure in the back seat. Paul then pulled out into a busy road and stopped at a line of traffic. As he glanced in the rear view mirror he saw a lorry bearing down on his car at what he thought was a considerable speed. In that moment, he thought to himself, 'The lorry's not going to stop; it's going to crush our car and Abigail will be killed.' As these thoughts were going through his mind, he felt the impact of the collision and saw the top of his daughter's head in the rear-view mirror. Some three months after the accident, he told me of his 'slow motion' recollection of each and every detail of the accident and of recalling two feelings – that of horror that Abigail might be killed, and the fear that he might never see her again. Although in Paul's mind the accident was horrific, the reality was that the lorry struck his car at no more than 16 km/10 miles per hour – no one was injured and the damage to the car mainly involved paintwork. Nevertheless Paul, a man with no previous history of mental health problems, suffered such a significant degree of PTSD that he only returned to work, following successful treatment, some six months after the accident.

To the outsider the accident involving Paul and Abigail was trivial. However, Paul's perception was far from trivial. The accident – in Paul's mind – threatened the death of his dearly loved daughter. In the days, weeks and months following the accident, Paul could not shift from his mind either the thought that Abigail could have been killed, or the consequences for his wife and himself had she been killed. His perception of the lorry bearing down on his car – apparently at great speed – was the central feature of his nightmares; his sleep was broken by these images.

An important matter that needs further exploration is whether or not people with PTSD perceive any sense of control over what is happening. It seems clear that most are experiencing events over which they have little or no control. On the other hand, one may often find that professional responders to accidents and similar events – police officers, firefighters, and paramedics and ambulance personnel – are less affected by horrific events because they are, in a sense, in control. For example, firefighters, when attending an accident and rescuing badly injured individuals from a car crash, have a specific job to do. Although they may be acutely aware of the pain and injuries of those trapped, they will be preoccupied by what they have to do in rescuing them from the wreckage. It is, of course, true that first responders such as firefighters will experience emotional reactions after horrific events and, over time, these emotional reactions may accumulate to produce PTSD or other identifiable psychiatric disorders. It is also the experience of professionals such as myself that the experiences of professional responders over time may lead to a vulnerability in such individuals and that, sometimes, they will react to an event in their own lives with a severe state of PTSD.

Traumas come in so many shapes and forms. Once more, there is a need to emphasize that perception of the individual experiencing the event is of considerable and central importance.

The case of Juliet

Juliet is an experienced paramedic who was stationed near a major motorway. She saw a large number of serious accidents resulting in death and major injury. Juliet was often involved, for several hours, in attending to individuals who were trapped in the wreckage of their vehicle. She told me some time later that she was nicknamed 'Miss Coolhead' by her colleagues because of the way she dealt with such events. However, one afternoon she was visiting her grandfather, a previously very healthy 85-year-old, in his own home. While she was standing in the kitchen with him, he suddenly collapsed and suffered a cardiac arrest. Juliet called for assistance immediately on her mobile phone and set about trying to resuscitate her grandfather with CPR. Although the emergency services arrived very quickly, all attempts to resuscitate her much loved 'Granddad' failed. Juliet suffered great shock at this tragic event and could not stop physically shaking. She was unable to sleep that night. Although her GP thought that being signed off from work would help her, Juliet remained in a state of shock and was then tormented by dreams involving scenes from accidents that she had attended over the years. She was also overwhelmed by a feeling of guilt that she had used CPR incorrectly on her grandfather. Despite reassurance from a number of individuals that she had done all she could, she blamed herself for her grandfather's death. By the time I saw her many weeks after her grandfather's death, she was unable to work because of her condition. She was having flashbacks involving memories of accidents she had attended. She lost a great deal of weight and one of the striking features in the way she presented to me was how trivial sounds from outside my room made her 'jump'. Juliet required several months of treatment before she could start work again, and the ambulance service for whom she worked greatly assisted her recovery by allowing a gradual reintroduction to her previous role, beginning with working a few hours a week in the control room and then step by step until she eventually reassumed her full 'front line' role.

The case of Juliet also highlights an important feature of many, but not all, cases of PTSD, namely the suddenness of the event. Often, traumatic events come without any warning whatsoever.

2

Types of trauma

The most common traumatic events seen by the average therapist or GP will be those associated with road traffic accidents, domestic violence and sexual abuse. Sadly, one also commonly sees victims of street crime – those who may have been assaulted by being punched and kicked and, too often, those who have been involved in stabbings and shootings. Less commonly one might see victims of natural disasters, such as earthquakes or volcanic eruptions. Recently colleagues have reported a number of cases of PTSD in the victims of flooding in the UK. These individuals had suddenly lost their houses and possessions and some had suffered a threat to their own lives or those of loved family members. I also know from my experiences in Australia that the many and all too common bush fires result in a significant number of cases of PTSD.

In recent years we have seen numerous cases of terrorist bombings and, of course, the recent decade has seen a great deal of war, causing untold misery to soldiers and civilian lives. In my own clinical experience I have seen victims of all these categories and also victims of major accidents involving mass transport, including the sinking of the *Herald of Free Enterprise* ferry off Zeebrugge in 1987, the King's Cross tube-station fire later that same year and the sinking of the *Marchioness* ferry on the River Thames in 1989.

One part of the UK that has been affected by continuing and widespread trauma is Northern Ireland where, over 40 years, including a period of 25 years (1969–94) when the Troubles were more intense, there have been numerous tragic events. In that period it is estimated that violence has caused the deaths of 3,600 people and more than 40,000 people have been injured, in a population of less than two million. Notwithstanding the peace initiative of 1994, the violence has continued, for example with the Omagh bombing in 1998. Various reports and studies have shown that 50 per cent of the population has had direct experience of the

11

Troubles. The PTSD of large numbers of them has been much complicated by alcohol and substance misuse (a very common feature of PTSD), and it is clear that PTSD and its attendant problems are now affecting several generations.

The differing nature of the trauma deserves some further comment. People who are victims of natural disasters are, in general, more accepting of what has happened, in the belief that one can do nothing about the course of nature and that a flood or an earthquake is, to put it one way, 'an act of God'. However, victims of crime, or those involved in accidents where someone else is clearly 'to blame', can often become preoccupied by anger towards the 'perpetrator(s)' – the person, people or corporation deemed responsible. This anger can often become all consuming.

Another aspect of being a victim because of the actions of others is the legal process that follows. Seeking some form of legal redress is, of course, understandable. Though no amount of money will restore life as it was, seeking compensation is very necessary – particularly if injury causes the loss of livelihood or, in the case of a child deprived of mother or father, there is a need to provide the child with appropriate care in the future. On the other hand, legal processes may be less than helpful because they often serve to act as a continual reminder of what has happened, so that the person is unable – to use a cliché – to 'move on'. In addition, the adversarial nature of law often means that even in the cases where the cause of the injury by one party has been clearly identified, there is often a denial of responsibility. Furthermore those who have physical and psychological injuries may be challenged by lawyers about the true severity of their condition. There is no intention in this book to dissuade anyone from seeking legal help or taking part in legal action. However, my years of clinical experience have shown that there is always a need to consider taking legal action very carefully with the assistance of a suitably skilled legal professional.

In the paragraph above I have used the word 'perpetrator' in the sense of the person or persons causing harm and possibly PTSD in another. However, perpetrators may also themselves have PTSD. One particular group of individuals has made a particular impact on me over recent years, namely members of the armed forces. I have seen a number of soldiers who have served in Afghanistan and

Iraq who have, in the course of their duties, been responsible for the death or serious injury of others. In some cases this involved armed individuals of 'the other side', but in one or two tragic cases the soldiers I have seen have been responsible for the death of civilians who became – to use an awful term – 'collateral damage'. The overwhelming emotion demonstrated by these servicemen has been guilt. I have frequently observed that these young men are often kind and considerate people who are simply unable to justify what they have done – although at an intellectual level they seem to accept the reality of a soldier serving in the theatre of war.

Another perspective involving perpetrators was identified in some research I undertook with others some years ago. We identified a number of research studies that showed that PTSD among prisoners was much higher than in the general population. Sadly, many of these prisoners had been victims of sexual abuse during childhood and then had gone on to commit crimes, often involving violence or sexual offences, for which they were imprisoned. Our research also identified a number of prisoners who had PTSD because of the crimes they had committed, notably a number of individuals, of previously good character, who killed another person in a fit of rage or under the influence of alcohol. While the prisoner population is not one that immediately draws sympathy from the general public, there are literally thousands of prisoners in the UK whose PTSD causes them untold suffering and distress. The prison health service does what it can within limited resources to provide treatment. However, in reality the majority of these prisoners will receive no real help at all for their problems.

One further group of those who have been traumatized deserves particular mention, namely those who have suffered childhood sexual abuse. This group falls into two distinct categories. First there are children and adolescents who present as deeply traumatized by recent sexual abuse and who may suffer a much wider range of manifestations than one sees in adults with PTSD. This book is not for them. In my opinion such children and adolescents require intervention by skilled professionals, with particular expertise not only in PTSD but also in treating children and adolescents per se.

The second category, who may be helped by this book, are those individuals who were sexually abused many years – often decades –

before. Many of these individuals are now coming forward as a result of the widespread publicity about high-profile cases. Some individuals – and I have now seen several such cases – who have come forward because of new police investigations, have identified themselves as victims of abuse many years before. The following case illustrates some of the issues involved.

The case of Irene

Irene presented to me at the age of 47, having been referred by her GP. She had been to the GP saying that she was becoming very anxious and depressed – she said that she did not know why – and that she needed to see someone with expertise in cognitive behavioural therapy (CBT), an approach about which she had read. The GP had known Irene for a number of years and knew that she had a history of mood problems and several episodes of self-harm. She had received very little previous psychological treatment, though she had been admitted to psychiatric hospitals on four occasions and also treated as an outpatient. However, from the notes that the GP had seen from the mental health services, it appeared that the central treatment approach used had been anti-depressant medication and some occasional sleeping tablets. The records showed that Irene had been diagnosed with several conditions, including mixed anxiety and depression, and a 'borderline personality disorder'.

When she came to see me, Irene told me that she believed she would benefit from psychological treatment, having read quite extensively about CBT. I went on to ask her about her thoughts and feelings and, quite spontaneously, she told me that her desire for psychological treatment had been prompted by a resurfacing of memories from her childhood. Indeed she told me that she had previously 'put these memories well behind me'. When I asked further questions it appeared that about a year previously there had been publicity about the abuse, many years before, of children in a particular home run by the local authority. One of the workers in the home had been prosecuted for the historic abuse of two particular children who had come forward and prompted a police investigation. Irene had read about the case in the newspapers, seen reports on the TV news and immediately recognized the name of the abuser and the care home where the abuse took place. Irene was then overwhelmed by memories of this particular care worker subjecting her to sexual abuse that took place over a two-year period when she had not yet reached puberty. Irene could not be certain about the timing of the abuse – she said that although she remembered the specific incidents, the rest of her memory of that time was 'something of a blur'. However, she thought the abuse occurred when she was between eight and ten years old. Irene went on to tell me that she had left the children's home when she was 15 and began working in a factory. She had found herself a room to live in and she told me that although her wages were very low, she was happy for the first time in her life. Following two years working in a factory, Irene took a number of other jobs and then evening classes to become a bookkeeper. She recalls trying to 'block out as far as possible' memories of her childhood and to 'get on with my life'. Irene met her husband-to-be when she was 20, and she told me that for the first time in her life she felt part of a family – he had a large extended family who were very kind and considerate towards her. Irene married at 22 and quickly became pregnant with her first child, a son. However, following the birth she became depressed, this episode being the first of many. Over the years Irene's episodes of depression became complicated by a desire to hurt herself, which she did by cutting her legs and abdomen. Although when she first met her husband she was able to embark on a sexual relationship, sexual intercourse was never pleasurable for her and she was never able to reach an orgasm. As time went on, Irene eventually refrained from any sexual activity, which caused her husband to feel alienated from her. Between episodes of depression and self-harm, Irene was able to regain a reasonable mood and continued working in an office for much of the time. Just after she became aware of the case of the abuser at the home where she was abused, Irene told me that she became overwhelmed by feelings of depression, self-loathing, guilt and that – for the first time in many years – she was experiencing flashbacks in the form of vivid images of her abuser and what had taken place all those years before. In order to attempt to cope with these feelings, Irene began drinking alcohol every evening, something she had never done before. Very quickly one or two glasses of wine became a bottle of wine a night. This was the time that Irene came to see me.

There were two components to Irene's treatment. The first was trauma-based CBT – more of this later in Chapter 4 – that focused specifically on helping her cope with the memory of those awful events of all those years ago. The second component comprised therapy aimed at dealing with the longer-term consequences of the sexual abuse – the low mood, feelings of loathing and guilt, self-harming behaviours and, of course, the need to deal with the escalating alcohol problem and to help her and her husband regain a sexual relationship.

Irene's story emphasizes the fact that the long-term effects of trauma, particularly exemplified in those who have suffered childhood sexual abuse, lead to very important life-changing consequences. Thus although Irene was able to push memories of the abuse 'to the back of her mind' and, in her words, 'get on with life', the trauma was causing the longer-term mood disorder and feelings of self-loathing and – when the trauma emerged – her problems with alcohol.

Irene, like others who have suffered the long-term effects of childhood sexual abuse, required therapy over a number of months to deal with both the trauma itself and the long-term consequences. Altogether Irene received 30 treatment sessions from me, in addition to some sessions from an alcohol therapist. She and her husband also went on to have some therapy to address the sexual and relationship difficulties. This therapy was successful in bringing the couple closer together. At the time of her discharge from my care, Irene still had some residual symptoms of depression but had abstained from alcohol for many weeks and was determined to remain abstinent for the rest of her life because the alcohol had made her problems much worse. Irene told me that she believed she was 'as well as I can get'. She appeared confident that she could now deal with the memories of the abuse, which occasionally occurred. Therapy had provided Irene with a range of coping mechanisms that meant, in her words, that she 'would not cave in or give up' as she had in the past.

In my experience there is no completely happy ending to cases such as Irene's. Psychological therapy and, in some cases, medication may be very helpful in restoring reasonable function and helping the person to achieve a more sustained and improved quality of life. Nevertheless it seems clear that there is no such thing as a cure because abuses that occur during childhood – particularly those that occur in the setting of the deprivation of a normal family – and over a long period of time, will never be erased from the memory.

Underlying mechanisms – the cause of PTSD

As we will see in Chapter 3, there are a large number of signs and symptoms of PTSD. However, what actually causes these is a matter that has preoccupied research scientists for many years. One way of looking at the causation of trauma is to consider the biological mechanisms that are put into place when trauma occurs. Simply put, a sudden threat to one's life or a sudden shock causes the body to react with an extreme 'fight or flight' reaction. The body is put into a state whereby it can react with the greatest efficiency. This entails the outpouring of adrenalin from the adrenal glands, placing the body into a state of preparedness for fight or flight. Thus all systems of the body go on high alert – pulse and blood pressure increase, rate of breathing increases, muscles become tense and the digestive system works rapidly to absorb as much nutrient as possible into the system. Simply put, everything in our body goes into overdrive. The fight or flight reaction is extreme, and in some cases individuals remain in this permanent state of biological preparedness. Thus many people with PTSD will – as in the case of Juliet noted in the previous chapter – remain jumpy and will react with a 'startle response' to even trivial sounds. Practitioners often see individuals sweating and shaking and, on taking their pulse or blood pressure, find that these are elevated above normal. The extreme fight or flight reaction may also lead to changes in brain chemistry, and these changes will involve alterations of the balance of chemicals that control mood and anxiety levels.

Over the past decade or so, scientists have used magnetic resonance imaging (MRI) scans to investigate PTSD. Studies have shown that the amygdala – a centre in the brain involved with fear – can become hyperactive after a traumatic event and thus set off false alarms. Similarly it appears that a centre in the brain – the hippocampus – responsible for memory and emotional experience may also be affected.

In parallel to the biological effects of trauma, the memories of events become deeply embedded in our memory banks, and these memories are of such significance that they tend to take a prominent position in all domains of thinking. These parallel processes, both biological and memory, become linked and then serve to interact with each other in a vicious cycle. Thus memories produce more physical manifestations of fight or flight, and more fight or flight produces an overflow of memories into consciousness and so on. It is these underlying mechanisms that then produce the signs and symptoms of PTSD. I am sure that the research scientists who, over the years, have worked so systematically and skilfully will find the model I have just described overly simplistic. It is true that what goes on in the brain and in our processes of thinking and memory is complicated and not entirely understood. Nevertheless

I think that it is important that people with PTSD are able to see that their symptoms are generated by a vicious cycle involving both mind and body. (Those interested in a more detailed and scholarly account should see the excellent review article by Jonathan Sherin and Charles Nemeroff (2011).)

3

Defining PTSD

For the past 30 years or so, psychologists and psychiatrists have attempted to define PTSD in a way that would be understood by any health professional. More recently those responsible for the psychiatric classification systems have made very welcome attempts to make these definitions as jargon free as possible. The English-speaking world has two classification systems available. First, published not only in English but also in other languages, is the *International Classification of Diseases* published by the World Health Organization (WHO). At the moment their classification system is being revised; the new system should be published in 2017. While the WHO system, currently known as *ICD-10*, contains a definition of PTSD, the system published by the American Psychiatric Association (*Diagnostic and Statistical Manual of Mental Disorders*, Fifth Edition – *DSM-5*), which was introduced in Chapter 1, is arguably the most clear and the easiest to follow.

In order to qualify for a diagnosis of PTSD using *DSM-5*, the person needs to meet a number of criteria. The first concerns the cause and requires the individual to experience one or more of the following:

- to directly experience the traumatic event;
- to witness in person the event as it occurred to others;
- to learn that the traumatic event occurred to a close family member or friend;
- to experience repeated or extreme exposure to details of the traumatic event.

The criterion specifically states that this does not apply to exposure to media, such as TV, films or photographs.

The second criterion involves the person persistently re-experiencing the event in one of the following ways:

- by thoughts or perception;
- by images;

- by dreams;
- by illusions or hallucinations;
- by flashback episodes;
- by intense distress or reaction to cues that symbolize some aspect of the event.

The classification also notes that children re-experience traumatic events in other ways, for example through repetitive play.

The next criterion to be met concerns avoidance of anything associated with the trauma and numbing of general responsiveness. In order to meet this criterion the person has to be doing one of the following:

- avoiding thoughts, feelings or conversations associated with the event;
- avoiding people, places or activities that may trigger recollections.

To meet the fourth criterion the person needs to experience two or more of the following symptoms involving thoughts and mood:

- inability to remember an important aspect of the event;
- persistent and exaggerated negative beliefs about self, others or the world;
- persistent distorted thoughts about the cause or the consequence of the event;
- persistent negative emotional state;
- markedly diminished interest or participation in significant activities;
- feelings of detachment or estrangement from others;
- persistent inability to experience positive emotions.

The fifth criterion concerns alterations in arousal and reactivity. The person needs to exhibit two or more of the following:

- irritable behaviour and angry outbursts;
- reckless or self-destructive behaviour;
- hypervigilance (constantly on the lookout for signs of potential danger);
- exaggerated startle response (jumpiness at the slightest sound or stimulus);

- concentration problems;
- sleep disturbance.

The classification system also states that in order to meet the diagnosis of PTSD there must be significant distress or impairment of function and that the duration of the condition must be more than one month.

In addition to the symptoms mentioned in the *DSM-5* manual, adult survivors of childhood abuse may commonly have additional problems, poor physical health and preoccupation with real or imagined worries that their abuser is still in the community and has access to children or young people. Many people who have suffered abuse during childhood struggle with parenting or relationships.

The classification system includes a helpful section on the manifestations of PTSD in children and describes the reactions of children of five years or younger. Typical reactions in these young children can include a fear of being separated from the parents, crying, whimpering, screaming, immobility or aimless motion, trembling, frightened facial expressions and excessive clinginess. It is also noted that parents may notice regressive behaviours – for example, when a previously toilet-trained child becomes incontinent.

The classification also notes that children between the ages of 6 and 11 show other signs – for example, extreme withdrawal, disruptive behaviour and an inability to pay attention. Children in this age group may also be affected by regressive behaviours, nightmares, sleep problems, irrational fear, irritability, school refusal, outbursts of anger and fighting with others. The classification also describes children possibly having physical complaints that do not have a medical basis, such as complaining of stomach ache.

There are a number of very helpful websites that set out the above information. Much of the description of the criteria given here is to be found in the Medscape website, a very useful resource for health professionals and the general public (<http://emedicine.medscape.com/article/288154-clinical>). This website has distilled the key information from the large *DSM-5* manual and serves as a very faithful reproduction of the diagnostic criteria.

One criticism of the criteria in the *DSM-5* manual is the failure to convey what many people describe as a great personality change in those with the more severe forms of PTSD. Many people who present for treatment recognize these changes in personality. In addition, family members and friends will often describe personality changes as the main manifestation.

One of the key behaviours that cause people to come to the conclusion that a personality change has taken place is the occurrence of angry outbursts.

The case of Dominic

At the time of his accident Dominic was a 25-year-old who had just married and whose wife had just given birth to their first child, a daughter. Dominic was working as a plumber in a block of flats that was being refurbished. One day he was working in an upper floor flat when the flooring collapsed. He fell 4.5 metres (15 feet), landing very awkwardly and feet first. He did not lose consciousness but was suffering great pain because of the broken bones in his legs and feet and various back injuries. Dominic was taken to hospital, where he stayed for three months, enduring a number of operations. He was discharged to a rehabilitation centre, with a great deal of metalwork inserted into his feet and ankles to hold his broken bones together. He was in much pain, which had not responded to the usual powerful painkilling medication. I saw Dominic several months after this, following the intervention of the solicitor who was providing him with advice about a claim against those responsible for not ensuring that the flooring was safe to work on. This solicitor had had a great deal of experience with people with PTSD and recognized that Dominic needed assessment and treatment for his condition. It was noteworthy that although Dominic had been seen by several orthopaedic experts to assess his physical injuries, none of them had identified his psychological problems. Unfortunately this is a commonly encountered scenario. Doctors who deal with complex physical injuries often do not take sufficient account of the psychological consequences. This may be because they are preoccupied about providing the best possible physical treatment or it may be because many doctors have not received sufficient training in the psychiatric aspects of physical conditions.

At assessment, Dominic presented as a very sad young man, who spoke at length about never being able to return to his previous life in which he played football, ran half marathons and was able to work long days in his job – earning a very good wage for his efforts. Dominic went on to tell me that he had flashbacks of the accident and, at night, was often woken up by dreams where he saw and felt himself falling and then lying on the ground, looking up. Sometimes he had other nightmarish dreams of subjects not connected to his accident, usually involving his being chased and then falling into water and struggling to breathe. He also told me that many reminders of his previous work triggered flashbacks in the form of vivid mental images of the accident and thoughts that he would never be able to work again. He told me that any TV adverts for DIY products could set off these flashbacks; likewise the sound or sight of ambulances or TV programmes about hospitals. Once I had completed my initial assessment, when Dominic told me of the wide range of symptoms that certainly qualified him for a diagnosis of PTSD, I asked to see his wife, alone. I first explained to her that Dominic had told me a good deal about his problems, and I asked her for her perspective. She immediately told me that Dominic had become 'unbearable to live with', adding: 'He's a right pig.' She also told me she was on the verge of leaving him. She told me that the mild-mannered man she had met, fallen in love with and married had undergone 'a massive personality change'. For no apparent reason Dominic would start to shout and swear at her and, more recently and on more than one occasion, had raised his fist to strike her – although he managed to restrain himself. He would then become tearful and apologetic, saying 'Why do I do this?' Dominic's wife told me that she was becoming very frightened of his behaviour. As the interview progressed it became clear that Dominic had hidden much of his distress from his wife and had not told her about his intrusive memories. He had also minimized the amount of pain he had endured, and she knew little of his very negative thoughts, which included a consideration of suicide.

However, his wife did know that Dominic had nightmares, and she told me that he would wake sweating and shouting but would not reveal the content of his harrowing dreams to her.

It became necessary to involve Dominic's wife in much of his treatment, and once he was able to share his experience with her he obtained some relief. His treatment included a number of strategies to help him cope and directly treat his PTSD; one of these was to teach him a range of anger-management techniques to help him control his irritability and anger.

The case of Dominic demonstrates another feature of PTSD, namely the need for treatment for this condition to take place alongside additional treatment for physical injuries. Surgical treatment, although necessary and eventually helpful, produces stress of its own. In Dominic's case he required several operations over the next two-and-a-half years, some of which led to periods of immobility because of the need to have his legs in plaster. It was thus necessary to ensure that psychological treatment and support took place alongside physical rehabilitation.

The classification systems are far from perfect, and within psychiatry and the legal profession there are critics of the diagnostic label. However, the vast majority of professionals will say that those who suffer trauma often present great challenges and the classification system provides a very useful way of guiding an assessment and providing a checklist of groups of symptoms that need to be considered.

The concept of nervous shock

Some readers of this book may have come across the term 'nervous shock' within the context of legal proceedings brought because of the negligent actions of others. Nervous shock denotes the effect of a horrific, sudden and usually life-threatening event on a person, leading to a definable psychiatric illness – such as PTSD. Nervous shock may apply either to a person who has directly experienced the event (known in law as the primary victim) or to someone witnessing the event (known in law as the secondary victim). Although the concept of nervous shock was introduced to clarify matters, like many legal concepts it has become complicated by judges, so that lay people and medical professionals alike are usually bewildered by the way it is applied in legal cases. The reason for including this topic in this book is because legal proceedings involving those with PTSD are nowadays quite common. My advice however is brief: ask the lawyer involved for an explanation!

How common is PTSD?

One of the striking findings of research is that only a minority of people who suffer traumatic events go on to have PTSD. Thus not all trauma turns out to be traumatic!

A range of research has been carried out across the world to establish just how many people suffer a traumatic event. Much of the research has involved populations in the USA, and as a number of the studies were large, it is reasonable to assume that the numbers identified are reasonably accurate for the USA as a whole. Furthermore, when one looks at the nature of the traumas involved (the sudden death of a loved one being the most frequent traumatic stressor in one study), it is reasonable to assume that the numbers identified in the research in the USA may be similar to those found in populations in other countries. Estimates produced by the research of the percentage of the population involved in traumatic events vary between 60 and 80 per cent for men and 50 to 70 per cent for women. However, these numbers are obviously greater than the numbers of people who actually develop PTSD – thus begging the question of why some people develop the condition and some do not. Although at first sight it may be surprising to see so many people witnessing or being involved in traumatic events in a lifetime, if one thinks about the subject more, most of us can recollect traumatic events such as accidents that we have seen or been involved in, the death of someone close to us and so on. If one thinks more widely about sexual assault – which is now known to be much more common than previously realized – and trauma occurring during medical treatment, one can begin to see that the research indicating that only a minority of the population are spared witnessing or being involved in a traumatic event is probably an accurate representation of life's realities. Think even more widely and ask the question of people living in war zones or near natural disasters – for example, the population of Northern Ireland who lived through more than a quarter century of the Troubles that touched so many lives, or those throughout the UK affected by the widespread flooding of 2014 – and one can begin to see that being affected by a traumatic event is not only frequent, but also beyond the control of all of us.

Who goes on to develop PTSD?

Estimates from research studies conducted across Europe, the USA and Australasia of people developing PTSD after a traumatic event range from 10 to 15 per cent for men and 20 to 30 per cent for women (remember that these percentages are of people who have experienced trauma – that is, percentages of percentages). Nevertheless, when one considers these figures within the entire population, the numbers involved are considerable – several million of the UK population, for example. Research shows that it is much more likely that PTSD will develop in people who have been assaulted, particularly victims of sexual assault, than people who have been involved in accidents and disasters. Once more, witnessing the sudden and unexpected death of a loved one comes very high on the list. As I have noted above, PTSD may be seen as developing as a result of a combination of biological and cognitive – meaning processes involving memory, perception and thinking – factors. Researchers have gone on to identify other variables that serve to maintain PTSD. It has become clear that various avoidance behaviours – such as avoiding any reminders, trying to suppress thoughts associated with the event or refusing to talk about it – may increase the likelihood of PTSD becoming a longer-term problem. In addition, some people seem particularly vulnerable to the biological processes that follow trauma, and PTSD can be seen in some as a chronic stress reaction, affecting individuals exhibiting high levels of physical stress in general.

In clinical work one comes across many cases where, prior to the traumatic event, the individual appeared to be psychologically very 'well adjusted'. Conversely, I have also come across cases where individuals deemed by others to be psychologically vulnerable do not go on to develop PTSD, even after a very serious event.

The case of Ruth

At the time of the traumatic event Ruth was 42 years old and had come to see me several times over a period of 15 years with quite severe anxiety symptoms, involving an avoidance of public places and most forms of transport. Due to her anxiety she had a greatly reduced social life, being unable to sit in the middle of a row in a theatre and finding parties and social gatherings very anxiety evoking. Over the years Ruth made some gains with treatment and, in many respects, she carried on a normal life, being able to work, marry and bring up two children. Family life was, in her own words, her 'sanctuary'. As a result of treatment, Ruth was eventually able to take a job in the West End of London, travelling there by underground. Just before the event that affected her, she had contacted me to say that she was enjoying her job but was finding the travel to work very stressful. Indeed she had had two panic attacks during which she thought she was going to die from a heart attack. I therefore arranged an appointment.

Two weeks later, on 7 July 2005, just before she was due to see me, Ruth was on an underground train when a terrorist bomb exploded. She told me that the sound of the explosion was deafening and that she initially experienced great shock. She then recollected hearing people screaming and shouting and it took some time for Ruth to be brought out of the train tunnel and back to the surface to be reunited, eventually, with her family. Surprisingly, Ruth did not develop PTSD as a result of her experience. She told me that quite soon after she had experienced the initial shock of the explosion she realized she was uninjured. She was reassured, and became convinced she would be rescued. Several other passengers also provided reassurance to each other and to Ruth, while they awaited evacuation. Although Ruth was aware that she was shaking, she recalls feeling an inner calm as she was led along the tunnel to safety. She came to see me three days after this event and I simply let her talk and tell me her story. Ruth was obviously very keen to resume 'normal' life and told me several times that she had gone to church to pray and give thanks that she was uninjured and that her life had been spared. I saw Ruth again on a couple of occasions in the next six weeks in the course of a process of 'watchful waiting' – a topic to which I will refer in Chapter 4. Although Ruth had some sleep disturbance and other symptoms of anxiety, in the longer term she appeared to be unaffected by PTSD, although her memories of the involvement in the tragedy will be with her for ever. Ruth subsequently told me: 'My prayers are with those who have lost loved ones and those who have been injured – my heart goes out to them.'

The story of Ruth illustrates that the causation of PTSD that requires treatment is still somewhat of a mystery. One could speculate that a number of positive factors prevented her from developing the condition. However, I do know that her story is by no means unique. Many individuals develop an initial stress reaction after a traumatic event, with symptoms that might be quite severe. These symptoms might include flashbacks, nightmares and panic attacks, but in many cases the stress reactions subside fairly quickly. This improvement often occurs within the context of receiving a great deal of support from friends and family, from other survivors of the same event or, in the case of Ruth, processes occurring through a particular religious faith. A number of research studies have also shown that some people develop PTSD after an horrific event, but that without intervention of any kind the condition eventually resolves over a period of weeks or months.

We do know that there are a number of important factors that appear to make PTSD more resistant to recovery. One of the most significant is the use of excessive amounts of alcohol or illicit substances (we will return to this topic, in particular in Chapter 7). There is, of course, an almost universal acceptance that in times of shock 'a stiff drink' sometimes assists. Therefore one can see how someone with a range of symptoms of anxiety, often causing great distress, will seek solace in alcohol or other drugs. We know from long-term studies conducted on populations of war veterans that the use of illicit substances and excessive use of alcohol makes PTSD not only resistant to treatment but makes it much worse. In turn we know that co-morbidity – the combination of PTSD and the misuse of alcohol or other substances – may lead to devastating consequences, such as the break-up of families and a life descending into crime and imprisonment. One can see from the story of Dominic that anger can become a very prevalent emotion in PTSD, and if one adds to angry feelings the use of illicit substances or excessive use of alcohol, it is easy to see how anger will develop into actual violence, with often devastating consequences.

Another factor linked to the longer-term development and maintenance of PTSD is, as noted above, the nature of the event and of someone being 'to blame' for its taking place. Thus it is common to see innocent victims of road traffic accidents becoming incensed when they see 'the other driver' either receiving a minimal sentence for his or her recklessness or not being prosecuted at all. The anger and resentment that follows may often serve as a maintaining factor. One also sees this phenomenon in people who have been traumatized by medical negligence. Unfortunately, many victims of proven medical negligence receive no apology in the immediate period after the negligent act – and may only receive one, grudgingly, several years later. In the meantime, they are unable to think further than the legal processes involved in trying to seek some restitution for the wrongs done to them through the negligence. As stated before, the decision to proceed with a legal claim is not an entirely straightforward matter although, conversely, it has to be said that doing so may lead to improvements in the practice of a particular hospital, and those affected may feel they have done something to stop similar acts of negligence happening to others.

Sex differences

One very notable finding across research studies is that female victims of traumatic events are at higher risk for PTSD than male victims. The reason for this is unknown. The available evidence suggests that these sex differences are not due to the higher occurrence of sexual assault among females, prior traumatic experiences or a pre-existing depression or anxiety disorder. Thus the mystery continues!

PTSD in children and adolescents

In recent years I have enjoyed the privilege of working with a number of inspiring colleagues at the National Drug and Alcohol Research Centre in Sydney, Australia. One of these colleagues, Dr Emma Barrett, has drawn my attention to the very substantial problem of PTSD in children and adolescents. Her work has identified research showing that 14 per cent of adolescents have PTSD, a percentage nearly twice that of the adult population. The problem is further complicated by the finding that half of these adolescents have co-occurring substance-misuse disorder. When one looks at this detail it is somewhat understandable that adolescents with PTSD may turn to illicit substances or alcohol – or both – to relieve their symptoms and, thus, self-medicate. What happens then is that the PTSD and substance abuse continue as a vicious cycle and, in many cases, all that becomes obvious to others is the substance abuse, the PTSD remaining largely undetected.

Substance abuse and/or the excessive use of alcohol in young people has significant neurological consequences because the brain continues to develop over teenage years and beyond. Young people who abuse substances or drink even modest amounts of alcohol often go on to demonstrate considerable problems with learning and memory. This vicious cycle in adolescents often leads to conflict with the criminal justice system because of crimes committed to sustain the use of substances or because of the outbursts of aggressive and violent behaviour that may be caused, either by the PTSD itself or the use of substances, particularly stimulant drugs such as the amphetamines. The team in which Dr Emma Barrett works – at the National Drug and Alcohol Research Centre – is leading the world in research on this topic and, at the time of writing this book, Dr Barrett and her colleagues are developing treatment methods that specifically target adolescents and are therefore rising to the challenge of treating both problems – PTSD and substance misuse – simultaneously.

Other psychiatric diagnoses that overlap with PTSD

Over the years the classification systems for mental health problems have been revised a number of times. One of the reasons for these revisions is the great overlap that exists between a number of diagnostic categories. In the case of PTSD there is often considerable overlap with a diagnostic category known as adjustment disorder. Adjustment disorders are, quite simply, psychological reactions to stressful life events. They are very commonly seen in populations who have lost their homes because of natural disasters or war-related events. Many life events, such as loss and bereavement, may also lead to adjustment disorders. These disorders come in different shapes and forms, and although most resolve within six months, some become chronic – particularly in the case of bereavement, where the source of stress is ongoing. Adjustment disorders will often present with considerable disturbance of emotion. It is therefore not uncommon to see people who are profoundly sad, have feelings of hopelessness, lack of enjoyment, feelings of anger or guilt, sleeping difficulties and difficulties with concentration. Additionally, many people with adjustment disorders have suicidal thoughts. It is also not uncommon for people with such disorders to have flashbacks in the form of vivid images. Therefore, in many ways, the more severe forms of adjustment disorder are, to all intents and purposes, the same as PTSD. In some cases the difference between one person with PTSD and another with an adjustment disorder rests with the person making the diagnosis. The difference in diagnosis may also be caused by the disorder being characterized more by a general disturbance of emotions rather than other symptoms, in which case some doctors and psychologists prefer the diagnosis of 'adjustment disorder, with prominent disturbance of emotions'.

Similarly, people who develop depression following a sudden bereavement may also demonstrate a range of symptoms indicative of PTSD. It appears that in such cases a diagnosis of depression is reached when the person presents with such a depressed mood that other symptoms, which may include intrusive memories, flash-backs and irritability, are – by comparison to the mood – secondary.

If you have been diagnosed with an adjustment disorder, or depression, but have many of the symptoms described in this book, you will find Part 2 particularly helpful, as the coping strategies described apply to diagnostic categories other than PTSD.

4

Professional treatment

How can I access professional help?

The first port of call for accessing professional help in the NHS is your GP. Your GP might then refer to the Improving Access to Psychological Therapies (IAPT) programme, where therapy from suitably trained therapists is available.

IAPT was developed as the government's response to a great shortage of suitably trained psychological therapists and, over the past six years or so, has been rolled out across the UK, with a varying amount of success. Some parts of the country now have a substantial number of suitably trained therapists; others have not done as well. People with PTSD will need to be seen by the so-called 'high-intensity' therapists. IAPT also employs 'low-intensity' therapists to treat less complex mental health problems, such as mild to moderate depression and general anxiety states. High-intensity therapists are professionals who have been provided with substantial training and who should be familiar with all the evidence-based approaches – that is, treatment approaches supported by research evidence – recommended by the National Institute for Health and Care Excellence (NICE).

Unfortunately, many people with PTSD and other conditions that require specialist psychological intervention have to wait weeks or months for assessment and treatment. Sometimes the GP would prefer to refer you directly to the clinical psychology service of the local NHS Trust, where therapies would also be available.

It is clear at the time of writing, and will probably be the case for some years to come, that there are barriers to receiving satisfactory treatment for PTSD within a reasonable timeframe. For that reason people often turn to the charitable and independent sector for help. Increasingly, for example, those who serve or have served in the armed forces are being treated by services set up by charities. In addition, the armed forces offer 15 regional rehabilitation units in the UK and Germany. While much of the emphasis of these units is on those who have had serious physical injury and require long-term rehabilitation, they have access to specialist psychological services. As I mention in Chapter 6, organizations such as Combat Stress offer treatments on either a residential or non-residential basis for those with PTSD. The NHS also provides specialist traumatic stress services. To find out whether there is such a service in your area, try putting the search terms 'specialist PTSD services, NHS' into an online search engine and you will find a list of specialist services. NHS Choices is a website (<www.nhs.uk>) that also offers a section on the treatment of PTSD; this explains how cognitive behavioural therapy (CBT) works and who might benefit from it (see the section 'Cognitive behavioural therapy for PTSD' later in this chapter). This part of NHS Choices also contains a short video clip by Professor David Clark, a world-renowned CBT expert.

If you receive specialist treatment for PTSD you will probably be referred to a therapist who is a clinical psychologist by background, a nurse therapist who has undergone specific CBT training or other health professionals who have received specialist CBT training.

In my opinion it is important that those receiving treatment for PTSD be seen by an individual who is appropriately registered, either with the British Association for Behavioural and Cognitive Psychotherapies (<www.babcp.com/Default.aspx>) or the Health and Care Professions Council (<www.hcpc-uk.org.uk/index.asp>). All psychologists are now registered with the Health and Care Professions Council. Accessing the above websites will enable you to identify the background qualifications of the practitioner.

If you are to access a therapist in the independent sector, it is important that you ensure that this therapist offers an appropriate evidence-based method of treatment. Your GP will normally have access to information about suitably trained individuals in your area. You might also make enquiries of your local independent psychiatric hospital – for example, one of the dozen or more Priory hospitals in the UK, hospitals run by Cygnet Healthcare or the Capio Nightingale Hospital Group. There are also other independent psychiatric hospitals in the UK. This book does not offer particular suggestions about services provided by the independent sector. However, the hospitals mentioned above all have specially qualified psychiatrists and therapists who would be well placed to provide CBT.

NICE guidelines

The National Institute for Health and Care Excellence (NICE – formerly called the National Institute for Health and Clinical Excellence) provides guidance, sets quality standards and manages a national database to improve people's health and prevent and treat ill health. NICE makes recommendations to the NHS on new and existing medicines, treatments and procedures and treating and caring for people with specific diseases and conditions. Its recommendations are also directed towards local authorities and other organizations in the public, private, voluntary and community sectors. As NICE guidelines are developed very carefully and are based not only on rigorous reviews of evidence but also on consensus opinions from a wide range of individuals with knowledge of and expertise on conditions, they must be at the forefront of the minds of those who provide – and indeed seek – treatment. The latest NICE guidance on PTSD was published in March 2005 and will be described below. This guidance – CG 26 – is due for review some time after 2015, but it is likely that any changes will be fairly minimal. It is possible there will be some updating regarding the range of medications that may be a useful treatment for PTSD. The reader should find the NICE website – <www.nice.org.uk> – helpful and relatively easy to navigate. The full guideline for PTSD is lengthy, but the website has available a very useful booklet of around 40 pages, *Post-Traumatic Stress Disorder (PTSD): The treatment of PTSD in adults and children* (full details are in the Further reading section at the end of this book), which is used extensively by health professionals and the general public. I recommend anyone with a particular interest in PTSD to read online or download and print off a copy of the booklet.

There are two very important points to emphasize about this particular guidance. First, NICE is very clear in stating that the initial response to trauma should not be to offer treatment immediately. It is particularly noted that, where symptoms are mild and have been present for less than four weeks after a trauma, 'watchful waiting', as a way of managing the difficulties presented by people with PTSD, should be put into place. What follows this period of watchful waiting should be a follow-up contact arranged within one month.

Watchful waiting is now recommended for a very wide range of medical conditions, as it has become increasingly emphasized over the years that, too often, we intervene unnecessarily. There are many examples in medicine of unnecessary interventions. For example, in the case of acute ear infections, doctors have in the past been too ready to prescribe antibiotics and anxious parents have added to the problem by pressurizing their family doctors to intervene. There is now a range of evidence that suggests that simple watchful waiting in such cases is more effective, with the advice given along the lines of:

> By all means, give the child some Paracetamol to reduce pain and temperature, but just allow nature to take its course and, in most cases, the infection will resolve; if symptoms become worse or do not resolve within a day or so, then of course more active intervention may be required.

Other examples of where watchful waiting may be indicated are cases of benign prostate enlargement and, indeed, depression. The author's own experience of clinical practice and research provides plentiful evidence that people – even with severe levels of depression – may recover without medical intervention. Time is, indeed, a great healer.

One particular example from my own clinical practice illustrates the point.

The case of Hannah

Hannah, at the time of the traumatic event a 25-year-old medical secretary, was working in a central London clinic. Since her teenage years Hannah had suffered from general anxiety and panic attacks and had visited her GP on a number of occasions. Her GP had often offered tranquillizing medication and antidepressants, which Hannah turned down. She decided instead to attempt to deal with her problem by taking lots of exercise and to lead a busy and challenging life.

It was for this reason that Hannah joined a local gym and, rather than finding work at a local hospital, decided to take a job in London, which necessitated a tube journey but paid a very attractive salary.

Hannah travelled home late, after 11.30 p.m., after going out with some friends from work. After she left the tube she went to the side street in which she had parked her car to make the short journey home. She used a side street as the station car park was quite expensive. As she opened her car door she was confronted by two men whose faces were hidden by balaclavas. They threatened that if she didn't hand over her bag and mobile phone they would knife her. She did what they said, but as she was handing the items over, one of the men kicked her in the leg and slapped her in the face. These men told her to lie down on the ground and then escaped. Hannah did not sustain any serious physical injuries, but was very shocked and distressed by her experience. She was taken to hospital and was discharged to be reunited with her family.

In the days after the event, Hannah remained in a shocked and upset state and saw her GP. Her GP telephoned me some ten days after the robbery to ask if I would see Hannah as an emergency. I arranged to see her soon thereafter. Hannah told me what had happened; during this account she sobbed and was clearly very distressed. She also explained that she had turned down the offer of sleeping tablets from her GP, although she was still experiencing very broken sleep and had had some nightmares about the robbery. Nevertheless, a couple of days before she saw me, Hannah had decided that she would return to work. Her employers were very sympathetic and told her to come in for a few hours only and go home if she felt she needed to. Although she continued to have very disturbing flashbacks of the event, she took the view that she would be better off distracting herself through her work. Hannah told me that she had received numerous messages from friends and colleagues offering support. Some of her friends also suggested that she should join them in distracting activities.

I took the view that watchful waiting would be the best strategy in her case, and arranged for Hannah to ring me in seven days' time for the purpose of checking out her progress. I also arranged a more formal appointment for her to come to see me at my consulting room. On the following day I received two telephone calls from Hannah's father, who was most concerned that I had not offered treatment, and one from Hannah's GP, who had received the fax that I had sent him saying that I would engage in a watchful-waiting exercise. Both Hannah's father and the GP wanted to know why no treatment had been offered when Hannah was still so upset by her experience. I simply reiterated what I knew about intervening too early and reassured them that, should Hannah's state change for the worse, I would be only too happy to revisit my decision.

A week went by and Hannah rang to tell me that she was feeling 'much better and stronger'. She told me that her employers had agreed a plan for her to work limited hours and build her working day, slowly, over a few weeks. At that time she also said that her experience had put into perspective her past anxieties and panic attacks, which she now saw as 'worrying over nothing'.

I did indeed see Hannah on the four-week anniversary of the robbery, and then some three months later. At that time Hannah still had upsetting memories of the event, telling me that she would never forget her experience. She told me that she found the first two or three weeks very difficult. She dealt with this by first of all having someone to meet her at the end of her tube journey and then gradually facing the journey home alone, but ensuring that she only used the car park at the station that was covered by CCTV, and when there were 'lots of people around'. She told me that she felt she needed to conquer the apprehension and distress that she suffered. Nevertheless she made a number of firm rules for herself about using car parks late at night.

This case history demonstrates how a process of watchful waiting is the best strategy for some. I really did no more than offer Hannah an ear to her story and to encourage all the things this young woman had already planned – going back to work, meeting friends and engaging in distraction. In a sense, despite her previous history of anxiety, a natural process of resilience and resilience-building took over.

In the summer of 2013 I received a postcard from Australia with a message from Hannah, saying:

> Just thought I'd let you know that the horrendous event has made me a stronger person. Very ironically, coming to Australia by aeroplane, on my own, is something I would have never done had it not been for being robbed and assaulted – however, I think my trust in others has really suffered and I now see risks in situations that I previously thought harmless. Nevertheless I'm not going to stop living my life.

Another example of how different people react differently!

The NICE guidance for PTSD also includes a 'Do not do' recommendation. It is specifically stated:

> Non-trauma-focused interventions such as relaxation or non-directive therapy, that do not address traumatic memories, should

not routinely be offered to people who present with PTSD symptoms within 3 months of a traumatic event.

(CG26, 1.9.1.8)

This recommendation does not negate the use of relaxation and similar approaches when used as an anxiety management strategy, in addition to a trauma focused intervention.

Also under the 'Do not do' heading it is noted that:

Drug treatments for PTSD should not be used as a routine first-line treatment for adults (in general use or by specialist mental health professionals) in preference to a trauma-focused psychological therapy.

(CG26, 1.9.3.1)

NICE guidance sets out the definition of PTSD, specifically mentioning that although it generally affects the person directly involved in the trauma or situation, it may also develop in members of the emergency services or in families of those involved in a traumatic event. The guidance emphasizes just how common PTSD can be, stating that it affects about 8 per cent of people at some point in their lives. The guidance emphasizes that the professional who treats the patient should provide enough information about the effective treatments for PTSD and about the condition. This recommendation, of course, forms part of the rationale for writing this book.

The guidance recommends two main modes of psychological treatment: trauma-focused cognitive behavioural therapy (CBT) and eye movement desensitization and reprocessing (EMDR).

Cognitive behavioural therapy for PTSD

What is CBT? One of the best answers to this question comes from Dr Judith Beck, of the Beck Institute in the USA. She says:

Cognitive behavior therapy is one of the few forms of psychotherapy that has been scientifically tested and found to be effective in hundreds of clinical trials for many different disorders. In contrast to other forms of psychotherapy, cognitive therapy is usually more focused on the present, more time-limited, and more problem-solving oriented. In addition, patients learn specific skills that they can use for the rest of their lives. These skills involve identifying distorted thinking, modifying beliefs, relating to others in different ways, and changing behaviors.

(Beck, no date)

Therefore CBT doesn't involve 'analysing' you; it doesn't subscribe to the theories of Freud and Jung; and your therapist doesn't ask you to lie on a couch while she/he discusses your unconscious.

In the process of therapy your therapist will work with you and find ways that you can help yourself.

The central components of CBT for PTSD include:

- helping the patient face up to memories of the traumatic event, which could involve assisting them in imagining the event and reliving it in the present tense, including all the thoughts and feelings associated with it;
- exposure to situations that evoke memories – in particular and where possible, helping the person visit the scene where the event took place;
- providing the patient with education about the nature of PTSD and, in particular, identifying factors known to increase problems, such as the use of drugs and alcohol, avoidance behaviour and so on;
- general anxiety-management training;
- engaging members of the family and/or significant others to assist in rehabilitation;
- dealing with any associated abuse of drugs and/or alcohol;
- developing coping strategies.

Although many websites will convey the idea that CBT is a recently developed treatment and has evolved from behavioural and cognitive psychology, the origins of CBT may be found in the writings of Greeks and Romans – such as Marcus Aurelius, the Roman emperor who provided cognitive behavioural advice on the widest range of subjects. More recently, as my much admired teacher Professor Isaac Marks pointed out to me many years ago, the philosopher John Locke (1632–1704) described what CBT therapists and psychologists call systematic desensitization, or exposure therapy, in his writings. Locke said, for example:

Your child shrieks, and runs away at the sight of a frog; let another catch it, and lay it down at a good distance from him: at first accustom him to look upon it; when he can do that, then to come nearer to it, and see it leap without emotion; then to touch it lightly, when it is held fast in another's hand; and so on, till he can come to handle it as confidently as a butterfly or a sparrow. By the same way any other vain terrors may be remov'd; if care be taken, that you go not too fast, and push not the child on to a new degree of assurance, till he be thoroughly confirm'd in the former.

(Locke 1693)

Thus some of our new ideas, described in scientific terms, are not all they seem and not really new!

Eye movement desensitization and reprocessing (EMDR)

EMDR was said to be first developed by a psychologist, Dr Francine Shapiro, when she noticed that certain eye movements appeared to reduce the intensity of the disturbing thoughts and images relating to the trauma. Dr Shapiro put forward the idea that traumatic images and memories overwhelmed normal coping mechanisms and were stored in an isolated set of memories (Shapiro 1989). Dr Shapiro developed a treatment that involved concentrating on an image linked to the traumatic event and related thoughts and feelings, while at the same time concentrating on external movements – usually the therapist's fingers. The treatment involves repeating this exercise for about 20 seconds and then attempting to 'let go' of the distressing memories. During treatment the therapist will encourage the patient to discuss the emotions experienced during the process. The treatment continues with an emphasis on changing the memories to more positive thoughts.

Over the course of treatment the patient is encouraged to seek out signs of bodily tension and, again, link these perceptions of bodily tension with positive thoughts.

A number of studies of EMDR have been conducted over the years, and the Cochrane Collaboration – an internationally recognized and highly regarded source of evidence reviews – noted that EMDR was as effective as trauma-focused cognitive behavioural therapy

(Bisson and Andrew 2007). However, it must be said that over the past two decades EMDR has been the subject of considerable controversy, many highly regarded experts arguing that the therapy worked through the exposure to traumatic memories (exactly as in trauma-focused CBT) and that the contribution of eye movements was irrelevant. Nevertheless, whatever the mechanism that leads to improvement, EMDR appears to be an effective treatment.

While psychological treatments are very strongly recommended, in addition to the 'Do not do' advice present in the NICE guidelines, there is particular mention of 'debriefing'. As the reader may know, following major disasters and the like, teams of counsellors and therapists tend to be dispatched immediately to 'debrief' disaster victims. There is now a range of research that shows that this 'debriefing process' is not very helpful, and indeed many victims of disasters feel much worse later, apparently because of the effects of debriefing exercises. What seems more important is for people to be offered practical support and information about how to cope over the following weeks, and that watchful waiting is the best strategy.

The NICE guidance has a specific section on children and young people. This makes some very helpful suggestions about the involvement of parents and guardians, making it clear that one should not rely solely on information from parent or guardian in any assessment, but should ask the child or young person separately and directly about his or her symptoms of PTSD.

Antidepressants in PTSD

It might be helpful here to say something about antidepressants, how they work and why they are used specifically in PTSD.

The history of antidepressants is interesting, as the first two classes of antidepressants were developed from drugs used to treat other conditions. The first antidepressants, discovered in the 1950s, belong to a group called the monoamine oxidase inhibitors (more usually referred to as MAOIs). These drugs were developed following the discovery that an antituberculosis drug, iproniazid, had a mood-elevating effect and patients in tuberculosis sanatoria were noted to display increases in mood, energy levels and appetite. Monoamine oxidase is an enzyme that breaks down various brain chemicals (notably serotonin, a neurotransmitter responsible for maintaining normal mood). Iproniazid was shown to act by inhibiting monoamine oxidase, thus maintaining reasonable levels of neurotransmitter substances in the brain (hence the term mono-amine oxidase inhibitor). Indeed it is one of the classes of drugs that are still recommended by NICE (see below).

The second class of drugs, also developed in the 1950s, was the tri-cyclic antidepressants. These drugs were developed from medications used as antihistamines in the treatment of allergy. Unlike MAOIs, the tricyclics improved mood, but had a beneficial, tranquillizing effect on anxiety levels. A further advantage of the tricyclic antide-pressants was the lack of any interaction with food – patients taking MAOIs should not eat a number of foods containing free amines. The most common foodstuff to be avoided is cheese, but there are others, including sedimented beers and wines, pickled herrings, some beans, meat extracts, some sausages and yeast products such as Marmite™. Eating these foodstuffs can lead to dangerous increases in blood pressure. For this reason MAOIs have been developed further and a new class of this drug, called reversible monoamine oxidase inhibitors, do not have these dietary restrictions.

The past three decades have seen the introduction of newer antidepressant medications, particularly the selective serotonin reuptake inhibitors (SSRIs). The most well-known of this group of medications is fluoxetine, more commonly known by its trade name, Prozac. Another class of drugs, serotonin-norepinephrine reuptake inhibitors (SNRIs), has also been developed. In addition to these two main classes of antidepressants, a number of other anti-depressant drugs, which also act on neurotransmitters, have been developed and marketed. These are called atypical antidepressants.

This book is not intended to provide a comprehensive account of antidepressant medication, and if you are prescribed one of these drugs it is important to follow your GP's advice and to read the leaflet accompanying your prescription very carefully. In general it is worth noting that all antidepressants – like all medications – have potential side effects. The side effects differ for each class of drug. The side effects of antidepressants generally tend to be worse in the first few weeks of taking the drug and then gradually diminish. In some cases patients will say that they experience no side effects in the long term at all. However, in consideration of side effects one needs to weigh up the balance of risks and benefits. Many people who have obtained great benefit from antidepressant medication will say that the side effects they have suffered are well worth putting up with for the longer-term benefits.

It is very important to emphasize that antidepressants do not really start to work until one has taken the medication regularly for approximately three weeks. Many of these medications only reach a peak of action after two to three months. If you embark on a course of antidepressant medication it is important that the medication is taken regularly, and one also needs to bear in mind that it is to be taken *as a course*, rather like taking a course of antibiotics. However, in the case of antidepressants, a course of treatment is often for a year or more (please also read my remarks a few paragraphs on about coming off antidepressants).

One question often asked is, 'Why do antidepressants work in cases of PTSD?' The answer is complex, and part of it involves the response, 'We don't really know!' Nevertheless there are several possible explanations. Many people with PTSD have very significant levels of depression, and it is reasonable to assume that regulating the mood chemicals in such cases may lead to benefits. Antidepressants are also of benefit in reducing anxiety levels, and some antidepressants are very useful in inducing sleepiness. Such antidepressants are therefore best taken at night.

Although we know that, in general, antidepressants do work well for some patients, they do not work well for others – why some respond and some do not is a continuing puzzle.

As noted earlier in this chapter (see p. 38), antidepressants are not recommended as a first-line treatment for PTSD. However, the NICE guidance specifically states that medications are indicated if the person prefers not to engage in psychological treatments or, importantly, should be used when he or she has gained little or no benefit from a course of such treatment. In the case of those who have a significant level of depression or high levels of anxiety, which may affect their ability to benefit from psychological treatment, medication is usually recommended.

The NICE guidance specifically states that particular antidepressants appear to provide most benefit. It specifically recommends two of the newer antidepressants (paroxetine or mirtazapine), as well as two older ones (amitriptyline and phenelzine).

As with treatments for depression, NICE guidance emphasizes the need to continue with medication for a lengthy period – it mentions 12 months before a process of gradual withdrawal from medication is indicated. It also mentions the need to provide patients with advice about side effects and discontinuation. There is a recommendation that antidepressants need to be introduced over a period of at least four weeks.

There is one continuing note of caution about the use of anti-depressants that needs particular mention. Some people have difficulty withdrawing from antidepressant medication once they have been on it for some time, and even in cases where the anti-depressant has produced significant benefit, it is now known that some people require weaning off the medication, a process that can take anything from one to several months to complete. Someone in this category would be advised by their GP to make very small reductions in dosage in a systematic way over a period of time. For this reason one should never stop taking antidepressants abruptly, and it is important that withdrawal be undertaken under medical supervision.

The NICE guidance is that if sleeping tablets are to be used, they should only be taken in the short term.

Other prescription drugs

NICE guidance is very clear about the usefulness of medication in the treatment of PTSD. However, I continually see, in my clinical work, patients who are taking prescribed medications other than those recommended in treatment guidelines. Many of these medications, in my opinion, may cause more harm than good. Although NICE guidance refers to the *short-term* use of hypnotic (sleeping) pills, I still see many people who are taking these regularly and have been doing so for months or even years. I also see people who are taking tranquillizers such as diazepam (Valium) and similar drugs (all in a group known as benzodiazepines), who likewise are taking them regularly – weeks, months or even years after the traumatic event. While it is certainly true that some patients require the use of such tranquillizers to deal with the immediate acute distress that follows a trauma, all the guidelines issued to doctors state that such medications should only be used in the short term. Similarly, I still see a small number of people who are prescribed a group of drugs called beta-blockers. These drugs, which are very effective in the treatment of high blood pressure, are used to 'damp down' the arousal levels of people with PTSD. They act by slowing the heart rate and reducing physiological arousal. In a textbook I edited more than 25 years ago (Gournay 1989), a review of the evidence concluded that beta-blockers were ineffective treatments for anxiety in the long term.

Why, then, are these drugs prescribed?

There are several answers to this question. One lies in wide-ranging evidence, accrued over decades, that doctors 'like to do their own thing' and base their judgements on what may be effective for a particular patient on matters unconnected with evidence of effectiveness. Some doctors will sometimes have their judgement swayed by seeing a person in great distress and realizing that a particular medication will lead to immediate relief of a specific symptom (benzodiazepine tranquillizers do work very well at first), although at the same time they may realize that long-term use may be positively harmful. Nevertheless, because of their human desire to relieve suffering, they may continue to prescribe the medication, and then the phenomenon of a 'slippery slope' is set in train.

What, then, are the adverse effects of these medications?

As mentioned above, the largest group of medications commonly used in people who manifest anxiety and sleeping problems are the benzodiazepines. The most popular of these groups of drugs is diazepam (Valium) and there are, of course, a number of very closely related compounds.

Valium is the drug referred to in the 1966 Rolling Stones' song 'Mother's Little Helper', which emphasizes the numbing and harmful effects of long-term use of the drug (the 'yellow pill' mentioned describes the 5 mg Valium tablet). Sadly the song's message of caution was not heeded for more than a decade. In 1987 there were, in the UK, 27 million prescriptions for benzodiazepines. Since then mental health services here and across the world have been trying to deal with patients who have become addicted to these drugs. There is no doubt that benzodiazepines do reduce or, if enough is used, obliterate anxiety. However, the effectiveness of anxiety reduction quickly diminishes and addiction takes over. There are now guidelines in place that tell doctors very clearly that these medications should be used only in the short term. Nevertheless, long-term prescribing of these medications still occurs. In the end, benzodiazepines are a bigger problem than the original problem prescribed for. Testimony to the widespread problem of their use is the difficulty patients have in withdrawing from them – many GPs will continue to prescribe because patients simply find the withdrawal process so distressing, and too rapid withdrawal may lead to dangerous reactions.

Sleeping tablets, prescribed in the long term, may lead to exactly the same problems as benzodiazepines. Indeed some sleeping tablets are simply benzodiazepines taken at night rather than during the day. The most popular sleeping tablets taken today in the UK come from the group known as 'Z-drugs' – for example, zopiclone and zolpidem. Although these are not benzodiazepines, the problems associated with long-term use are similar. Both benzodiazepines and Z-drugs are now known to cause particular problems in the elderly, notably concerning balance and mobility and a range of others concerning memory and thinking.

All the above drugs, benzodiazepines and Z-drugs, interact with alcohol, and the results of the interaction include excessive sedation, an increase in memory and thinking problems and, in some cases, behavioural disturbance including outbursts of aggression.

In conclusion, therefore, sadly there are many people who are receiving prescription drugs not recommended by NICE. Moreover, some of these drugs are universally known to cause significant problems if taken in the long term. Should you be receiving any of these drugs, other than in the short term, you should first of all look at the NICE guidelines and, armed with these, go to your GP or the doctor who prescribed the medications, saying that you have read the NICE guidelines and in particular mention that they state that tranquillizers and sleeping tablets should only be prescribed as a short-term measure. It may be that your doctor has a very good reason for prescribing such medications, and I believe that it is very important that you are able to discuss these reasons with your doctor and satisfy yourself that the medication you are taking will be beneficial in the long term, rather than harmful.

A useful website providing information on the short-term use of benzodiazepines is <www.bupa.co.uk/individuals/health-information/directory/b/benzodiazepines>.

For people dependent on benzodiazepines a helpful website – and one I and several of my GP colleagues recommend to patients – is <www.patient.co.uk/health/stopping-benzodiazepines-and-z-drugs>.

There are also a number of self-help groups for those dependent on benzodiazepines – <www.benzo.org.uk> provides comprehensive information about self-help and self-help groups.

NICE guidance – support for families

The guidance has a specific section on support to families and carers, recognizing that PTSD will have a considerable impact on family members and others. The guidance specifically states that the family should be provided with information about PTSD and that families and carers should be informed about self-help and support groups. In addition to this guidance it is worth emphasizing that families and carers will often need to be provided with specific advice while the person with PTSD is receiving treatment.

5

Older people and complex cases

There is no age at which PTSD ceases to be a problem. One needs to remember that older people may have PTSD as a consequence of seeing a much-loved spouse suddenly die; as a result of an event linked to medical treatment; or – and this is a sad indictment of our society – because they have been the victim of crime.

The case of Daphne
At the time of the crime, Daphne was 85 years old but still enjoyed a great deal of independence. She had been widowed some 10 years before, following 50 years of very happy marriage. Daphne lived on her own and was fortunate insofar as she had a loving relationship with her son and daughter, who lived close by. Both children had children of their own and, altogether, Daphne had five grandchildren, all of school and university age.

Daphne enjoyed various activities, including a lunch club for older people, going to a book club and attending a keep-fit session at the local gym once a week. She also drove her car to visit friends, although she limited herself to local trips. She did most of her own shopping as she realized that relying on online shopping would deprive her of the exercise entailed in walking to the shops. She also enjoyed the social interaction that took place with shopkeepers she had known in her local town for many years.

On one such shopping trip Daphne went to a cashpoint to withdraw some money. As she turned around, after taking her money from the cash dispenser, she was confronted by a man who snatched the notes she held in her hand and punched her on the side of the face. Daphne fell to the ground and remembers experiencing a searing pain in her arm, which later proved to be a broken bone. She then recalls lying on the ground, sobbing. A number of people quickly came to Daphne's assistance and she was taken to hospital, where she was X-rayed and treated for a broken bone in her arm and severe facial bruising. In addition Daphne lost one of her remaining teeth (she wore a partial denture), and the inside of her mouth was swollen. Although she did not lose consciousness she was advised to spend the night in hospital under observation, and she recalls that every time she attempted to close her eyes to rest she had vivid images of the man's face and felt intense terror. Daphne was eventually given some diazepam (Valium – a minor tranquillizer) and was able to sleep, albeit somewhat fitfully, for a few hours overnight. In the morning, at her own insistence, Daphne was discharged from hospital to the care of her son and daughter-in-law, who took her to their home. Over the days and weeks that followed Daphne remained in a state of shock and sobbed for much of the time. Her son recalls her repeating over and over again, 'Why did he do this to me?' Additionally, Daphne continued to experience sleeping difficulties and some nights was awoken by nightmares, the content of which she couldn't recall. She declined the offer of more tranquillizing medication, because it made her feel 'groggy'. After about six weeks she said that she was feeling less nervous and decided that she wanted to return to her own home (where she had lived for 50 years), but within half an hour of doing so she was overcome by the fear that someone might break into her house. She also felt unable to go out on her own, although while she had been staying with her son she had been able to visit the local town in his and her daughter-in-law's company.

Daphne was then referred to the local mental health services for specialist treatment. Daphne was seen by a psychiatrist who formed the view that she was one of those individuals who should be offered some medication as a short-term measure to help her sleep. Although initially Daphne was very reluctant to take this, she accepted a course of sleeping tablets at a low dose, to be taken every night for one week, every other night for a further week and then discontinued.

In addition the psychiatrist who saw Daphne referred her to one of the community psychiatric nurses (CPNs) assigned to the team working with older people. This particular CPN had received some training in CBT and had experience of caring for victims of crime.

The CPN called on Daphne the next day so that she could see for herself what Daphne's living arrangements were like, the better to understand her day-to-day activities – the healthcare term is 'activities of daily living' (ADLs) – and obtain a picture of how the trauma might have affected them. She also spent over an hour listening to Daphne's account of the robbery and subsequent events. Over the next week or so Daphne, with her son, daughter and their spouses, had several sessions with the CPN, who advised that the best plan would be to attempt to build up Daphne's confidence very gradually by helping her to take small steps towards regaining independence. The CPN also told Daphne that every time she saw her she would focus on the trauma and

its effects. She provided Daphne and her family with a range of information about PTSD, including some printouts from the very informative
website, NHS Choices. The CPN emphasized the need for Daphne to
return, as much as possible, to her previous activities. She explained
that this should be achieved in steps, and that Daphne needed to face
situations that might initially cause anxiety.

One of the practical measures the CPN arranged was to provide
Daphne with an alarm button, which she wore on a cord attached to her
clothing. This alarm button would therefore enable Daphne to summon
help if required. The first step in helping her regain independence was
for her to return to her own home but to have her daughter sleep in
the second bedroom, so that Daphne felt more secure at night. By this
time the plaster cast on Daphne's arm had been removed and she now
felt sufficiently confident to be able to go to her dentist to have some
restorative dental work carried out. Over a period of several weeks she
was able to return to some level of independence – for example, to
resume her lunch-club visits and keep-fit exercises. However, everyone
agreed that she would never regain sufficient confidence to return to her
previous level of independence and, when she needed cash, she did this
with the assistance of another person. Daphne required six months of
intervention from the CPN, who saw her weekly for about three months
and then gradually reduced the frequency of her visits.

This case history demonstrates some important aspects of PTSD. First
and foremost, it can occur in any age group. The second aspect that
requires emphasis is that one needs to take into account the age of the
person involved. While there is specific guidance on PTSD and treatment in adolescence, there is nothing to guide health professionals
in its management in older people. In Daphne's case she required
a number of measures specifically related to her age, including the
provision of an alarm – many older people who live alone wear such
alarms. It was also important that the health professionals involved
in Daphne's care were those with some experience and expertise in
dealing with older people with mental health problems. Finally, the
age of the individual does have some bearing on the targets to be
achieved. At her age Daphne could look forward to many more years
of life (bearing in the mind that the number of people reaching their
centenary is increasing apace). However, despite improvement in
longevity, age brings infirmity and a slowing down of physical and
mental processes. Daphne was fortunate in having a loving family

who lived nearby; many older people are much more isolated and may require a great deal of help from voluntary and statutory services. In my experience this help is available, but one needs to know where to look. Victim Support is a charity that works with the police and other agencies and can provide very important information and advice – see <www.victimsupport.org.uk>. Similarly, the mental health services for older people are also an important resource. In some people's minds these services only provide care for those with dementia. This is not the case. Indeed services for older people will provide care and treatment for those with depression, anxiety and other mental health problems. Such services are comprised of doctors, nurses and other health professionals who have particular experience and expertise with older people and thus provide treatment and care that is age appropriate and will take this into account when designing treatments.

The treatment of complex cases involving physical injuries

The vast majority of articles, chapters and books on PTSD fail to deal with the co-existence of significant physical problems in people who also have high levels of PTSD. Anyone who sees large numbers of people with PTSD will know that the presence of physical injuries and their consequences are almost the norm. I have described the case of Dominic (see Chapter 3), who exemplifies the presence of serious injury alongside PTSD.

In the case of road traffic accidents, one of the most common problems is whiplash injury. Although it is a colloquial rather than medical term, 'whiplash injury' is used by many doctors to describe the mechanism of the injury – the 'whipping' of the cervical spine. This mechanism leads to pain and stiffness in the neck and back and often other symptoms such as pins and needles and headaches. In mild to moderate cases of whiplash injury there are often no clear findings on investigation – for example, MRI scans often detect no clear abnormality. It is not uncommon, however, to see people who appear to have only sustained mild to moderate whiplash injury continuing to complain of considerable levels of pain and discomfort for months or even years after an accident.

In any average year I will see, in those presenting with PTSD, one or more individuals who have had a leg amputated, several individuals who have undergone numerous orthopaedic operations to pin, plate and fuse various bones and limbs, and many who have spent days, weeks or months in hospital. In addition to these individuals I will also see people with brain injury. These injuries range in severity. There are individuals who have lost consciousness for a few seconds and then gone on to suffer concussion and then possibly other consequences such as headaches and irritability that go on for weeks or months. At the other end of the spectrum of severity are individuals with such significant brain injuries that they will suffer long-term problems of memory, learning and concentration.

In addition to people with obvious physical injuries, if one works with a population who have been victims of sexual assault one will come across individuals with problems so distressing that they have not discussed them with their GP or any other doctor. Sexual assault often causes injury to intimate parts of the body and may, even in individuals who have not been physically injured, lead to ongoing serious problems relating to sexual function.

Why is the topic of co-existing physical injury and PTSD so important in a book like this?

The answer to this question is fairly simple: the physical and the psychological are inextricably linked. An individual's PTSD, which is caused by the original trauma (putting the body into a state of overwhelming fight or flight), will be much more complicated if that person also has to contend with significant physical injuries and their consequences. For example, take the case of a young man or woman – such as Dominic in Chapter 3 – who has never really had any significant physical illness and who has always enjoyed a very active lifestyle, taking part in sports, outdoor activities and so on. One can only imagine how such an individual will feel if, following an accident, he or she needs to have a leg amputated or numerous operations over months or years to deal with broken bones, damaged joints, torn ligaments and tendons. Even without any PTSD, someone in this situation would probably become, to say the least, fed up and miserable about their state and have great difficulty adjusting to a state of long-term disability. If one adds in PTSD, one can see how a vicious cycle will develop. In my experience one cannot separate the physical rehabilitation that some people need from the psychological. It seems to me to be fairly pointless to focus on treatment for flashbacks and the other symptoms of PTSD if one does nothing about helping a person adjust to their long-term disability. Ideally one needs to co-ordinate all treatment efforts. However, in my experience, carefully co-ordinated treatment, where physical and psychological approaches are drawn together, is the exception rather than the rule. In some cases where the cause of an injury is not in dispute and where an insurance company may pay for treatment, there may be funds available to employ a care co-ordinator whose central job is to draw together all the strands of treatment and conduct continuing-needs assessments.

One common problem I come across is the patient with a significant level of pain. Although, as I mention in several places in this book, physical exercise and increasing levels of activity are important strategies for efforts aimed at recovery from PTSD, unfortunately people whose activities are limited by significant levels of pain are compromised because they may be unable to undertake much exercise and may be greatly limited in respect of increasing activities. One therefore needs to adapt the advice that is provided so as to meet the needs of the individual. In my opinion it is essential that whoever is conducting psychological therapy communicate regularly with those responsible for physiotherapy, occupational therapy and other approaches for physical rehabilitation. And in reality those with PTSD also need to make sure that all those involved in their care are kept informed of all developments. Therefore it is important that those with PTSD receive copies of all reports and letters – this is a basic right – so that they can see what is being said. In turn, where there are several professionals involved, it is important that all relevant information is shared.

One other problem that arises in the cases of serious injury with accompanying significant pain levels is the matter of analgesic medication (pain relief). Some patients require long-term treatment with very potent analgesics, often opioids (morphine-like substances). While effective for the management of the pain itself, these drugs may make the patient sleepy, less active and, due to the way the drugs act on the central nervous system, possibly more depressed than normal. Some drugs of the opioid category, used long term, may cause panic attacks and increased levels of anxiety.

Pain interacts with the symptoms of PTSD to produce a worsening of both conditions, in a vicious cycle. PTSD leads to an increase in muscle tension, an increase in muscle tension will worsen existing pain and, of course, a worsening of pain leads to further psychological distress. Constant pain leads to depression, and we know from research that people with depression experience pain to a greater degree than those without.

In many cases patients with significant levels of pain will benefit from the pain management programmes available within the NHS. These usually involve input from consultant anaesthetists, who may give very helpful advice about different medications and special techniques such as 'nerve blocks'. The programmes usually have input from specialist psychologists, who will provide advice about psychological methods of coping. Occupational therapists (OTs) may also provide advice; their particular expertise is in the matter of dealing with problems related to activities of daily living (ADLs). OTs will also assist with occupational rehabilitation, housing needs and a range of practical matters.

One final topic worthy of mention is the matter of people who have suffered such traumatic brain injuries that they have problems with concentration, memory, attention and learning. One obviously needs to adapt any psychological approach to this group of patients. In such cases it is always helpful to have the input of a clinical neuropsychologist. The NHS employs a number of these specially trained psychologists, usually in brain-injury rehabilitation units but sometimes in other services. These individuals are psychologists who have been trained in a range of broad clinical skills, such as methods of assessing and treating problems like anxiety, depression and PTSD. However, they will also have received additional extensive, specialist training in the assessment of neurological problems and have been trained in the use of so-called neuropsychological assessment instruments. There are now a range of psychological tools that identify the way thinking and memory are affected in brain injury, and the results of the assessments may be very helpful to a clinician such as myself when it comes to designing a programme. At a very simple level, it may be necessary for me to see such a patient for brief consultations, so as to ensure that difficulties in concentration and attention are taken into account. It is also important to ensure that instructions to the patient are recorded or carefully written down, to take account of memory problems.

Where does all this take us in our understanding of PTSD and its treatment?

In a book such as this it is impossible to provide a comprehensive account of the many combinations of PTSD with various physical injuries. In turn it is also impossible to provide a truly comprehensive and exhaustive account of treatment approaches. However, it is important for any reader of this book to know that specialist services for people with a combination of physical and psychological problems are available within the NHS, with resources such as pain-management clinics and brain-injury rehabilitation clinics.

As with other matters of health, should you wish to discuss anything raised in this section of the book, the first port of call should be your GP. Your GP will have access to information about specialist centres within the NHS or, if this is indicated, within the independent sector. In my opinion the one, central matter that needs attention is the drawing together of various treatment approaches and the need for one person to have an overview of the care and treatment provided. I know from my own experience that many GPs will do this as part of their role as a primary-care family doctor and, to re-iterate, your GP should be your first port of call.

Part 2
HOW TO COPE WITH SYMPTOMS

6

Learning and talking about PTSD

Part 2 of this book is devoted to methods that people with PTSD can use to deal with some of the common manifestations of the problem. It is intended that this book is for use on its own for people who for one reason or another are not in receipt of professional treatment. However, the book is also intended to be used as a helpful addition to professionally delivered therapies.

It is my opinion that if you have had PTSD for a period of months or more and the problem has an effect on your life (your daily functioning, personal relationships and/or your work), then you should seek advice from a health professional. As I have said before, the first port of call is obviously your GP, who may be able to refer you to a suitable NHS professional who has the necessary skill and experience to help with PTSD. If you have not already done so, you should consult Chapter 4 on the NICE guidelines to familiarize yourself with the treatments that are effective and that may be offered.

You may find there is some overlap between the following chapters on coping with various PTSD-related problems. This is because some methods of coping are applicable to more than one problem. Please don't be surprised if you find some repetition!

Know what you are dealing with

In my opinion the first step one needs to take in the process of recovery is to learn as much as possible about your condition. I urge you therefore to consult Part 1 of this book if you have not already done so, since it outlines the main facts about PTSD and its treatment. It is essential to recognize that PTSD comes in many shapes and forms and that there can be a wide range of symptoms. Everyone is different, and in my experience some suffer more from one symptom than from another. Thus reliving the original trauma may be the most prominent symptom for one person; it may be nightmares for another; and yet another may experience an overwhelming sense of guilt about some aspect of the problem. Some people benefit particularly from sharing their experiences with others who have the same problem, and one cannot overstate the value of self-help groups. This, however, is a generalization – some people are simply not 'joiners', and find mixing in groups difficult if not positively aversive.

In addition to what is in Part 1 of this book, there are several organizations that provide very helpful information about PTSD and that also have interactive websites, where experiences may be shared.

- Mind (<www.mind.org.uk>) offers very helpful information about PTSD, and you may download a booklet about the condition and its treatment. Additional useful resources can be found on the websites of other organizations. For example, Combat Stress (<www.combatstress.org.uk>) is specifically aimed at people who have served in the armed forces. It offers not only information but also treatment and support services that are free of charge, employing highly skilled professionals who have provided treatment and support to literally thousands of veterans.
- For those whose PTSD follows the loss of a child or after a stillbirth there are several supporting charities. SANDS (<www.uk-sands.org>) has a network of support groups across the UK. Similarly, The Compassionate Friends (<www.tcf.org. uk>) provides a range of support to the bereaved. From my own experience I know that many bereaved parents and families suffer many of the symptoms of PTSD, including the reliving of painful memories and upsurges of various emotions, including anger, guilt and extreme anxiety.
- Another helpful charity is Assist Trauma Care (<www. assisttraumacare.org.uk>), which provides treatment based on NICE guidance (see Chapter 4).
- For adults who have experienced childhood abuse, the National Society for the Prevention of Cruelty to Children (NSPCC) has a free helpline (see the Useful addresses section at the end of this

book). This can also be used if you are worried about a child. *Any* worry about a child *must* – I emphasize *must* – be reported. Always much better safe than sorry. The NSPCC also has a very helpful website with specific advice on this topic: <www.nspcc.org. uk/help-and-advice/worried-about-a-child/online-advice/adults-abused-in-childhood/adults-abused-in-childhood_wda87228. html>.

- Other charities offer specific assistance with anxiety disorders and may be very helpful in providing help and support for those with PTSD who specifically experience panic attacks and general anxiety. Two in particular offer UK-wide services: Anxiety UK (<www.anxietyuk.org.uk>) and No Panic (<www.nopanic.org. uk>) both offer continuing support, via helplines.
- The NHS Choices website is also helpful in providing a range of useful contacts (see the Useful addresses section at the end of this book).

Obtaining information about PTSD and about the treatment and support services available is therefore an important first step. In my opinion it is also important that those close to someone with PTSD are also provided with as much information as possible so that they may better understand the condition.

Talking about it

Now we come to the need to 'Talk about it!' However, this is not always easy, and sometimes needs to be done with a professional rather than a family member or friend. It's important to be careful about selecting whom to talk to. Some people will never understand and simply don't 'get it'. Others may themselves become upset hearing you talk about the traumatic event. So the selection of the appropriate person is often difficult. Please do not feel that you don't deserve to talk about it. You do! Don't think that if you try to forget about it it will go away. PTSD is something that sometimes does diminish over time without any treatment, but one of the reasons it diminishes may be the fact that the individual is able to talk it through with an appropriate person.

One strategy that may be helpful is to write down your story. My advice is to do this in stages. Write down one account, then look at this and fill in detail. Leave the account for a day or two, read what you have written, then start all over again. Keep this process going, filling in details as you go. You will probably find this process upsetting, so take your time. Leave it for a while if it causes you to get too upset – but keep at it!

Most people these days like to use a computer or a smartphone for writing their story, particularly because these make editing easier. However, there's nothing wrong with good old-fashioned pen and paper.

Some people benefit from describing their story in picture form – in sketches or in paintings. It doesn't matter if you're not a world-class artist; if you think drawing or painting will be helpful, then do it. Expressing your feelings is the priority. Sometimes people benefit from making recordings. These can be made on your smartphone, on a Dictaphone or by video.

In my experience the putting together of a story on paper, or on a computer, in pictures and drawings or, in some cases, by poetry can be therapeutic in itself. However, it is usually helpful to share what you have produced with another person. In the course of my professional treatment of patients I usually ask them to write their account as well as telling me in our treatment sessions. I always ask my patients to repeat the writing-down exercise regularly, recognizing that each time the task is attempted, the emotions and feelings flow out. Quite simply, one recognizes that this particular form of therapy has ended when writing down or recording the story no longer gives rise to the release of unpleasant and distressing feelings or emotions.

7

Coping with avoidance and other problem behaviours

Avoidance is a common and central feature of PTSD. People with PTSD will develop avoidance behaviours whereby they avoid some or all of the situations that remind them of the trauma – and sometimes such behaviours can develop considerably. Thus, for example, people who have been involved in road traffic accidents will often avoid travelling past the scene of the accident or sometimes avoid driving completely. Others may not avoid driving but will avoid travelling as a passenger because they are not 'in control'. Such avoidance reactions may continue to spread, so that people who have been involved in road traffic accidents who avoid driving, or being conveyed as a passenger, may also avoid being conveyed in any form of transport – buses, trains, underground or aeroplane. Even walking down the street can be a problem for some people, and they may walk as far away from the kerbside as possible because of fear of being involved in an accident. Other people go further and will avoid any trigger involving transport accidents, namely TV programmes, reading newspaper articles and so on.

Please remember that avoidance is a very common response and is understandable, because avoidance behaviours develop to protect one from very painful memories. Avoidance reactions may include shutting off your mind to any thoughts connected with the trauma – sometimes simply thinking about the trauma will bring back intense feelings of fear and shock. This may set off a prolonged reaction, involving other emotions.

The case of Emma
Emma had been married for two years when she discovered that she was pregnant for the first time. Like all parents to be, Emma and her husband were thrilled at the prospect of the arrival of a new baby. They decorated their spare bedroom as a nursery, bought baby clothes and a

pushchair and other baby equipment. They told all their friends about their expected new arrival. Emma, who was working as an auditor in a large financial firm, decided that she was going to take a generous amount of maternity leave and asked her mother and mother-in-law to assist with childcare when she went back to work, at the same time making enquiries about having a part-time nanny.

Emma had an uneventful pregnancy, apart from some early morning sickness that abated after 12 weeks or so, and feeling tired in the second part of her pregnancy. However, from 30 weeks until she finished work when she was 37 weeks pregnant, Emma felt well and full of energy. Just after she finished work, at 38 weeks, Emma's waters broke and, following the advice of her community midwife, she waited until her contractions were fairly frequent before going to the hospital. When she arrived at the hospital she was examined by a midwife and then a doctor and it quickly became clear that there was a major problem, as both midwife and doctor were unable to detect any heartbeat. Emma and her husband reacted to this news with great shock, as all antenatal checks had been perfectly normal and Emma had felt her unborn baby move just a few hours before her waters broke. Sadly, Emma delivered a stillborn daughter some hours later. To this day, despite a post mortem, no one has discovered the cause of Emma's daughter's death.

Very understandably, Emma was in a state of great shock and described feeling numb following this tragedy. She was discharged from hospital but could not face going home to the house where the nursery had been prepared. She instead went to stay with her mother. Other family members were helpful insofar as they were able to remove all the items prepared for the baby's arrival. However, Emma still felt unable to return to her house for several weeks. Initially she did not want to see anyone apart from her husband and her parents, and she stayed in bed for lengthy periods. She had many of the symptoms of PTSD, including having vivid and distressing dreams of the events at the hospital. She expressed feelings of guilt that she should have recognized that something was wrong with her pregnancy. These feelings of guilt persisted, despite reassurance from doctors that stillbirths sometimes occur for no reason that can be determined, and that there is nothing that one can do to prevent such tragedies. Many friends and relations tried to contact Emma to offer their condolences, but she avoided all contact with them.

After six weeks Emma decided she should go out with her husband to do the food shopping, but on entering the supermarket the first thing she encountered was a young mother with her baby. Emma ran back to her car and went home.

Although Emma was eventually able to see one or two close friends, she avoided any discussion of what had happened and although her husband tried to encourage her to talk about her feelings of loss, she was unable to do this. Indeed Emma displayed considerable irritability and feelings of anger, and on occasion vented angry feelings towards her husband, without any particular trigger on his part. Emma's employers contacted her, having been told of events by her husband. Their approach was very sympathetic; they simply said she was to take as much time as she needed to recover and that she should return to work if she wished in graduated steps. However, Emma knew that two women in her office were shortly due to give birth and for this reason she decided that she could not return to work to face a situation with 'news of births and healthy babies', and told her husband that she was going to give in her notice. Her husband persuaded her not to do this.

It was at this point that Emma was referred to me for assessment, so that I could decide with her whether she should embark on a course of psychological treatment. At assessment, Emma's overall presentation was one of considerable sadness, and over the four, long consultations that followed, she was able to begin to tell me about what had happened to her and about a very wide range of emotional responses. She told me later on that this was the first time she had 'really opened up', and although she found it very difficult to do so, she had recognized herself that avoiding talking about the tragedy and her emotions was something she needed to tackle. Being able to talk to me then led to Emma's talking to her husband and, as she told me, 'opening up to someone she loved'. Emma was then able to see that talking was beneficial, and after our fourth consultation she told me that 'getting it all off her chest' led to a sense of relief. In addition to helping Emma with strategies to deal with other aspects of her PTSD, she agreed with me that tackling avoidance behaviour was a priority. However, she realized that this needed to be tackled in graduated doses of difficulty. She and I discussed a plan for breaking down her avoidance behaviours in a systematic way. As homework, Emma went away and wrote down all the avoidances she had engaged in and arranged these in a hierarchy, so that the 'easier to manage' avoidance behaviours were at the bottom and the 'most difficult to manage' at the top. At the top of Emma's list was visiting a work colleague who had just given birth to twins and being able to cradle one of the babies in her arms. At the bottom of the list of avoidance behaviours was the task of looking at pictures of babies on the internet. In the middle of the list was the task of going to the supermarket on her own, having undertaken a preparatory visit in the company of her husband and looking out for mothers and babies. Emma realized that all these tasks, aimed at exposing her to previously avoided situations, would cause her some distress. However, she realized that in order to begin rebuilding her life, this was necessary. Indeed she found many of the exposure tasks difficult, but once she had accomplished them she reported feeling much better. A very important aspect of Emma's exposure was the development of a return-to-work plan. With her permission, I first of all spoke to a member of the human resources department at Emma's firm and then to the firm's occupational health advisor. Emma and I negotiated a return-to-work plan over a period of three months, so that she began working a few hours a day for three days a week and then building up, eventually returning to work on a full-time basis. Returning to work involved further exposure to some of the situations she had avoided, particularly speaking to colleagues who had just returned to work themselves after the birth of children.

At the time of writing, Emma and her husband have decided to put on hold trying for another child. They feel that Emma needs to recover fully from her PTSD, and although it is several months since she began treatment, Emma still has some anxiety and periods of sadness. Treatment has, therefore, been reasonably successful. Emma realizes that a new baby will not, in any way, replace the daughter whose life was lost just before birth. She and her husband still grieve for their daughter, who was buried in a local cemetery and whose grave they visit every week to lay flowers.

The experience of stillbirth is much more common than one might realize. In Emma's case, the cause of the stillbirth was never known – it is only identified in about 40 per cent of cases. In the western world approximately one in 160 births are stillbirths. These rates are of course much higher in some other parts of the world. Stillbirth is the cause of a great deal of PTSD and, sadly, many women who might benefit from treatment do not receive it, partly because the PTSD is not recognized as a problem. In addition, many women who suffer from the emotional consequences of stillbirth go on to have other children. The needs of the living children are put first and so the emotional pain of the mother is sometimes obscured, although it may remain indefinitely.

As in the case of someone like Emma, one needs to have a plan for dealing with avoidance behaviours. In the case of those who have developed avoidance behaviours following accidents, it is sometimes important for them to receive the help of a co-therapist. A co-therapist – a family member or friend – can be enlisted to embark on a process of exposure. Thus someone whose PTSD has developed as a consequence of an accident may, with the assistance of the co-therapist, face travelling along various routes – in graduated doses of difficulty. In many cases it is beneficial to revisit the original accident site, and although this may be very depressing, this strategy is usually extremely effective in reducing distress.

In summary, it is important to recognize that avoidance of situations, thoughts or feelings only serves to perpetuate the PTSD, and such avoidance can lead to more avoidance behaviour, so that one's life can become extremely restricted. I also need to repeat that dealing with avoidance behaviour will cause distress in many cases. Therefore tackling avoidance behaviour needs to be undertaken in graduated doses of difficulty. One rule of thumb is that exposure tasks should be difficult for you, but manageable. If the exposure tasks become unmanageable, you have tried too hard and perhaps too soon. If this is the case, stop and replan your exposure. If the distress continues or gives rise to feelings or emotions that you consider to be overwhelming, please speak to your GP or – if you are receiving professional treatment – your therapist.

Coping with emotional numbness/depersonalization/ dissociation

Most people that I see after a particularly traumatic event complain that they feel 'numb'. Often this numbness fades after the traumatic event. In a way, numbness is a protective response – following the traumatic event and the shock that follows, the brain simply shuts down emotions to protect you. What often comes with the feeling of numbness is one of unreality. You may walk around feeling that you are in a dream. Due to numbness and unreality you may be unable to connect with other people. Many family members or friends comment that a person in such a state appears to be cold, uncaring or aloof. What often goes on in the mind of a person in this state of numbness is a preoccupation with themselves and, often, a fear that the way they feel is a signal that they are going mad or about to lose control. One word often used now in connection with these experiences is 'dissociation'. Dissociation can be defined as a detachment from one's surroundings and, in its severe form, may include detachment from any physical and emotional experience. Most of us have experienced mild dissociation in some shape or form. Such states are usually temporary and are often described as 'daydreaming'. In very severe cases, dissociation will be so overwhelming that the individual will not have memory for various events in their life.

As I have noted above, numbness and the accompanying dissociation often diminishes over time. However, where it persists it often presents as a very significant problem. First, people realize that they are not 'emotionally right' and, as previously mentioned, feel they are going mad or about to lose control. It is important for people experiencing such feelings to know that emotional numbness, detachment and dissociation not only generally improve with time but can be helped with a number of coping strategies. In Chapter 11, I will discuss 'mindfulness', a particularly helpful approach for feelings of numbness. Mindfulness is a meditation technique that helps one concentrate and focus on the present and on everyday phenomena. A simpler technique for diffusing feelings of numbness and detachment is the practice of slow breathing and concentrating on breathing in and out and on your senses. I often recommend a 'quick fix' breathing exercise, available – free of charge – on a podcast of the Mental Health Foundation, at <www.mentalhealth. org.uk/help-information/podcasts/stress-relaxation-quick-fix/>.

While these techniques are helpful as coping exercises, it is essential that one deals with the core problem – the trauma itself – and that the person experiencing emotional numbness is provided with an appropriate trauma-focused CBT or EMDR treatment, which were discussed in Chapter 4.

Drugs and alcohol and PTSD

This is such an important and complex topic that it is difficult to know where to start. We have known for many years that people with PTSD will use non-prescription drugs or alcohol to deal with their mental pain. Although reports of this phenomenon are associated with recent wars from Vietnam onwards, there are numerous accounts of the combination of PTSD and alcohol use in the Ancient Greek and Roman literature. Alcohol is perhaps the oldest anxiolytic (anxiety-reducing drug), and most would realize that it can provide temporary relief. However, many people turn to alcohol and/or various substances and then go on to develop such a problem that their addictions become the most prominent feature of the picture. There have been a number of research studies on the frequency of drug and alcohol problems in people with PTSD. These have revealed differing rates of occurrence: estimates of problem drinking or substance abuse vary from 10 per cent to 80 per cent, depending on the study consulted. To some extent they show that frequency of drug and alcohol problems depends on the nature of the trauma itself. Suffice to say, alcohol and drug abuse and addictions are very common in people with PTSD. In my experience these problems are often hidden from professionals such as myself.

At the beginning of this book I made specific mention of Northern Ireland and the widespread trauma there, related to the Troubles. Recent reports have drawn attention to the way large numbers of the population have 'self-medicated' their PTSD with drugs and alcohol. In turn, the evidence is clear that much of the problem has been hidden from health professionals, often because those with PTSD have little or no insight into their issues, particularly those who struggle with controlling drug and/or alcohol use.

The presentation of alcohol problems varies in people with PTSD, as it does in those without it. Some with PTSD report drinking in binges, which may relate to trying to deal with exacerbations of intrusive memories. Sometimes, however, alcohol use is characterized by a gradually increasing frequency and quantity of use, so that alcohol dependence sets in and, if one attempts to stop drinking, one develops withdrawal symptoms.

There seems little doubt that alcohol use makes the symptoms of PTSD worse. Although alcohol is a very effective drug for providing relaxation and a reduction in anxiety, the effects are short lived. If one takes more than a modest amount, what then follows, after a short period, is a mood of depression and irritability. In turn there are problems with sleep, and other difficulties increase. In its own right, excessive alcohol use can cause the onset of panic attacks and other features of anxiety, which were not present before.

One very helpful way of determining if you have a problem, or the level of the problem, is the use of the Michigan Alcohol Screening Test available on the internet at no charge – see <www.counsellingresource.com/lib/quizzes/drug-testing/alcohol-mast/>. Alternatively, a universally used self-test is FAST, which detects whether drinking is hazardous. This is a four-item questionnaire that asks:

1 how often you have had eight or more drinks;
2 how often in the past year you have been unable to remember;
3 how often during the past year you have failed to do what is normally expected of you because of your drinking;
4 if a friend or relative, a doctor or other health worker has been concerned about your drinking or suggested that you cut down.

Details of this questionnaire can be found at <http://alcoholism.about.com/od/tests/a/fast.htm>.

The substances used by people to help them cope with their PTSD depend to a certain extent on availability. Sadly, drugs of abuse are widely available and some that can be harmful in the case of PTSD, such as cannabis, are gaining increasing public approval. In different parts of the world the laws concerning drug use have been greatly relaxed.

Professionals in my line of work face the difficulty of making a correct assessment of the extent of alcohol or substance use in those who come to us for help. We are therefore in their hands and need to depend on their honesty in telling us what substances they use, how much they use and what effects they have. Sometimes the matter of honesty is not entirely straightforward because people have ways of denying the extent of the problem to themselves – particularly those who are developing alcohol dependency problems. In PTSD the dissociation and numbness often impairs the individual's insight.

What, then, does one do about dealing with an alcohol or drug problem? My own opinion, which has been informed recently by considerable involvement in a very important initiative funded by the Medical Research Council of Australia, has led me to the firm view that one needs to deal with PTSD and any drug or alcohol problem in an integrated way. Simply telling people to get help for their alcohol or drug problems before they can receive treatment for PTSD used to be a very common approach by mental health professionals. However, in my view this is not to be recommended and may deter people from seeking further help. What one is doing by recommending this approach is potentially removing from individuals their main method of coping with the problem – albeit one that is ineffective – without providing them with any solutions.

There may be a case for offering some short-term intensive treatment for alcohol or drug problems, for example short periods of residential treatment to detoxify in cases where physical health is poor or where there are withdrawal problems. In the case of alcohol addiction this intensive treatment may take place over a week or so. In this period it may be necessary to give vitamins and medications to keep serious withdrawal problems such as seizures at bay. However, where possible, people should be provided with treatment on an outpatient basis. In the case of alcohol problems, sometimes anti-craving drugs can be used; these are usually prescribed by specialist drug and alcohol services. Similarly, it may be necessary to obtain specialist help for coming off street drugs such as heroin or related compounds. Addiction to benzodiazepines, such as Valium, is common because these drugs are now widely available for purchase on the street or online. Addiction to benzodiazepines requires professional treatment and, if you are dependent on these drugs, the only way to deal with that is to seek treatment from the local drug and alcohol service.

What, then, are the self-help methods?

The first piece of advice is, if possible, to abstain completely from any alcohol or non-prescription drugs because these will inevitably make the PTSD worse. In the case of people who use alcohol, but not to the extent that this causes significant problems, cutting down over a few days and then stopping is the best way forward. However, if you are unable to do this despite all good intentions, then there is clearly a problem and you need to seek professional help either via your GP or the local drug and alcohol services that are available in all parts of the UK – contact details are readily available online, in libraries or via GP surgeries.

You might wish to attend one of the widely available self-help groups, such as Alcoholics Anonymous (AA) – <www.alcoholics-anonymous.org.uk> (see the Useful addresses section at the end of this book); tel. 0800 769 7555. Details of how such addiction self-help works is outside the scope of this book, but it is worth noting that AA meetings are freely available, cost nothing and, as the name implies, are strictly anonymous. AA offers 'open meetings' to the general public – anyone can attend.

A number of other resources in the voluntary sector are well worth exploring. Addaction, for example, which began in 1967 as an association of parents of addicts, is now a major service-providing charity staffed by professional paid workers and volunteers, and manages projects around the country. Its activities include:

- managing projects and services, including for a growing number of health authorities, social services, probation services, the prison service and police forces;
- helping drug users, their families and friends with support in working towards drug-free lives;
- information and support for children, parents and carers;
- training for professionals;
- community groups;
- services for homeless drug users;
- influencing policy and contributing to the debate around drugs and drug-related issues;
- organizing conferences and meetings.

NHS Choices also offers a range of information and advice about services. The website also contains very helpful video clips – <www.nhs.uk/livewell/drugs/Pages/Drugshome.aspx>.

Coping with sleeping problems

Sleeping problems are an extremely common consequence of PTSD. You need to remember that PTSD causes very high levels of physical arousal, and in such a state it is very difficult for the body to relax and for sleep to take over – even if you are feeling very tired. In addition, sleeping problems can be caused by the intrusive dreams and nightmares that are another common manifestation.

Although the symptoms of PTSD may subside over time, sleeping problems often become prominent. There are several reasons for this. First, people with PTSD often develop sleeping habits that are 'unhealthy'. Thus broken sleep at night may be followed by sleeping in until the late morning. Alternatively one might take oneself to bed for a prolonged period during the afternoon so as to 'catch up' with lost sleep. In addition, some people try to deal with the sleeping problem by drinking excess alcohol. Even in small quantities, alcohol can be disruptive to the sleep cycle. While you may fall off to sleep quickly after a few drinks, if you already have anxiety you will most probably wake a few hours later in a tense and anxious state.

As we have mentioned before, some people become reliant on sleeping medications, and when one tries to withdraw from these, rebound sleep problems may often follow. People with PTSD will sometimes develop distracting techniques that prove unhelpful in initiating and maintaining a good sleeping pattern. They may have a TV in their bedroom and hope that they can 'drop off' while watching a programme. For many years, research evidence has demonstrated that any sleeping problem requires one to attend to some simple rules of 'sleep hygiene'. The rules are as follows:

1 It is very important to try to stick to a regular habit and, in particular, to get up at the same time every day. With regard to going to bed, you should only do so when you are ready for sleep. This might mean, in the first instance, that with a waking time of 7.30 a.m. you do not feel sleepy until 2 a.m. or 3 a.m. Thus it might be quite difficult in the early stages to stick to this routine. However, if you can do this, a natural sleep cycle will eventually follow. Remember that if you set a particular bedtime, you will then begin to anticipate it and think about the problem of falling asleep. It is therefore much better to wait until a feeling of sleepiness takes over.

2 It is important to use common sense and to avoid caffeinated drinks such as tea and coffee in the evening and also to avoid alcoholic drinks completely.

3 It is also essential that you do not take any naps during the day or try to catch up on sleep. This will again require some effort –

if you have any degree of sleep deprivation you will have times during the day when your eyes may begin to close. Such times will follow particularly heavy meals. It is therefore important that you do not overeat and, if necessary, rather than eating a large lunch or evening meal that you eat little but more often.

4 With regard to distractions in the bedroom, it is important to try to reserve the bedroom for sleep only; trying to fall off to sleep with the TV or radio playing will be unhelpful in the long term.

5 If you cannot fall off to sleep within 20 or 30 minutes it is important not to stay in bed and toss and turn. Tossing and turning will in itself cause you to waken more. It is better to remove yourself to another room and engage in a distracting activity – nothing too exciting though – such as doing a crossword, knitting or simply reading the newspaper. Involving yourself in other more alerting activities such as playing computer games or attempting to solve problems in your life will not be helpful.

6 In the evening, simple relaxation exercises or having a bath and trying to relax will often aid sleep.

7 Physical exercise is useful for many people but you need to find out the best time of day to undertake this. Sometimes vigorous activity two to three hours before you go to sleep may be very helpful because of the degree of relaxation that follows. However, some people find that physical exercise will make them alert for several hours to come. In this case it is worth trying to exercise early in the day. Nevertheless, it is important to emphasize that exercising is a very helpful general strategy for dealing with sleep problems.

8 It is worth keeping a sleep diary recording how much sleep you get, when you wake up and how refreshed you feel. You may find that there is a link between what you record in your sleeping diary and what happens during the day – there may be particular triggers that lead to a disrupted sleep pattern at night and you might therefore be able to modify these triggers.

Remember to stick to these rules of sleep hygiene and eventually a much improved sleep pattern will follow.

I will set out in Chapter 11 further information about mindfulness, exercises for breathing and relaxation, and physical exercise.

In my opinion it is important that you try to develop your own pattern of using these approaches. For example, one person may find breathing exercises the most helpful strategy; another may find they result in no particular, positive change. However, it is my advice that you try all the methods.

I also recommend reading Fiona Johnston's *Getting a Good Night's Sleep* (full details are in the Further reading section at the end of this book).

8

Coping with panic and anxiety

Panic and anxiety are very common manifestations of PTSD. To cope with these problems, first of all it is essential to know what you are dealing with. Therefore, back to basics!

To begin, it is important to say that anxiety or fear is normal. Everyone, even the 'coolest' person, has anxiety sometimes. Worry and anxiety are part of the human condition. These feelings are experienced in all cultures, although some of the outward signs of anxiety vary across them. Having abnormal levels of anxiety, such as occurs in PTSD, can very simply be defined as a condition in which fear grows to proportions where the problem causes distress to the individual and upsets or interferes with his or her normal activities. It is also important to say that 'normal' fear has a survival function. When one thinks about it carefully, fear protects us every time we set out to cross a road or enter dark and unfamiliar surroundings. Thus, in the case of PTSD, the traumatic event produces an exaggerated 'survival response'.

Coping with hypervigilance

Hypervigilance, sometimes called hyperalertness, is one of the central features of PTSD. Others may observe hypervigilance in you when they see you jump at everyday sounds or react to everyday events with fear, as if something awful is about to happen. PTSD produces hypervigilance because the traumatic event has told you very clearly that you are in danger. The problem is that because people with PTSD who experience hypervigilance continue to think they are in danger, their bodies remain in a state of preparedness. You may feel that simply leaving your house is unsafe, and hypervigilance will be increased when you go into any situation that reminds you of the traumatic event. Thus for the victim of a road traffic accident, roads and traffic situations increase his or her level of preparedness. Those who have suffered an event in the street – a robbery, for example, or being knocked down on the pavement – may find themselves continually looking out for signs of danger and for people who could provide assistance, such as police officers. Many people with PTSD will begin checking arrangements for future events before they undertake journeys. Some take the extra precaution of having a member of the family or a trusted friend nearby at all times. When one talks to family members about their experience of travelling with someone with PTSD, they will often tell you that as a passenger, that person will put their foot on an imaginary brake or may engage in continual checking of the mirrors. Of more concern, they may shout, 'Look out!' to the driver, thus putting all concerned in real rather than imaginary danger.

The increased physical arousal that underpins hypervigilance can cause a wide range of physical symptoms, such as nausea, actual vomiting or diarrhoea. Those with hypervigilance also report difficulties in breathing, feeling very hot or cold, and palpitations.

Hypervigilance is therefore a very common consequence of being traumatized. However, you should remember the following: hypervigilance leads you to scan the environment unnecessarily for danger, and because of your state of trying to look at everything at once, you may actually miss really important signs of danger in the environment. The state of constant arousal will make you feel tired and cause you to have difficulties concentrating. This may actually lead to more risk of accident.

What can you do to cope with hypervigilance?

Bear in mind that hypervigilance is caused by a heightened state of arousal and having a body and mind on constant alert. It is therefore important to address both body and mind in developing coping strategies. I will describe below three methods to help you deal with hypervigilance.

To deal with the body first, acquiring techniques of relaxation, which I discuss in Chapter 11, is very important. In my experience, different methods of relaxation suit different people, and you should therefore experiment. One important matter that concerns all methods of relaxation is that of the acquisition of the relaxation skill. Relaxation skills need to be learned, and one can only learn through practice of particular techniques. Listening to a relaxation CD once will not give you this skill, although it may provide some temporary relief. In my experience, to acquire this skill you will need to practise your particularly favoured relaxation technique two to three times a day and to do this every day for perhaps several weeks. It is also my experience that people get bored with practising one technique only, and it is therefore advisable to try two or three different ones and to alternate them.

Physical exercise, which I also discuss in Chapter 11, is also helpful because, quite simply, exercise burns off arousal. Anyone who has completed 45 minutes' training by running, rowing, swimming, cycling or brisk walking will tell you that they feel more relaxed for it. As with relaxation, exercise needs to be practised regularly – at least four times each week – and it may take several weeks before you begin to obtain significant benefit.

Finally, to help with the mental side of hypervigilance, I recommend trying to acquire skills in mindfulness meditation. I also provide more detail about mindfulness in Chapter 11. Essentially, it is a method that allows you to concentrate and focus on the present and to notice the relevant – and sometimes beautiful – features of each day rather than trying to find danger wherever you are.

The nature of anxiety

Having now established that fear is normal and leads to certain physical and psychological responses, it is important to consider more systematically the nature of anxiety states. One very helpful way of looking at anxiety is to see it as three sets of systems that are present in a greater or lesser form and interact with each other, often called the 'vicious circle of anxiety' (see Figure 1). These systems are:

- cognitive
- physiological
- behavioural.

Cognitive

'Cognitive' simply means anything to do with thinking – thoughts, attitudes and beliefs. Thus one cognitive feature of anxiety is worry: the person who worries incessantly about trivia; the person who worries about what will happen tomorrow and in the more distant future; the person who worries about whether there is enough money in the bank to pay the bills; the person who worries whether the bus will be on time so that they won't be late for work. Put in this way: it might be said that we all worry, and this is true; however, worry becomes a problem when it is disproportionate to the thing that we are worried about. For those with PTSD there is often a general increase in worry. Anxiety disorders are underpinned by attitudes and beliefs, which are part of the personality structure of the individual. Thus someone with PTSD will usually show an exaggeration of previous personality traits, for example becoming even more obsessive about safety and engaging in excessive checking behaviour.

Physiological

Hearts beat faster when confronted with danger – there is not a person in this world who does not know this feeling. However, if our hearts beat faster and we break into a cold sweat at the sight of a harmless spider, this physiological response is disproportionate to the stimulus – the harmless spider – and therefore a problem (unless you live in Australia, where some spiders are far from benign!). In PTSD, all our body systems are in a state of constant alert and therefore, in addition to a fast-beating heart, muscles become tense, the intestines become overactive and much, much, more! In the extreme, anxiety can peak into panic attacks, which I discuss further just below.

Behavioural

All of us have a tendency to avoid the unpleasant. Because avoidance becomes particularly problematic in PTSD, I will be devoting a section to this topic (see 'Behavioural activation' in Chapter 9). Thoughts and feelings, physiological responses and avoidance behaviours build into a vicious cycle, and over time the general level of anxiety in people with PTSD becomes embedded in their daily life.

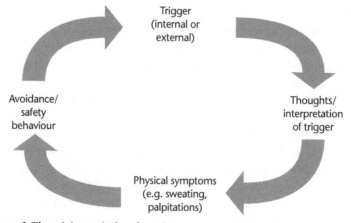

Figure 1 The vicious circle of anxiety

Panic attacks and panic disorder

Panic attacks are very common in the population. A range of research studies have shown that up to one in three people will have experienced panic during their lifetime. Thus in any one year millions of people in the UK will have panic attacks.

The American Psychiatric Association's *DSM-5* manual, which I discussed in Chapter 3, sets out the following list of panic symptoms, and states that one needs to experience four or more of them to qualify for the diagnosis of a panic attack:

- palpitations, pounding heart or accelerated heart rate;
- sweating;
- trembling or shaking;
- sensations of shortness of breath or smothering;
- feelings of choking;
- chest pain or discomfort;
- nausea or abdominal distress;
- feeling dizzy, unsteady, lightheaded or faint;
- derealization (feelings of unreality) and depersonalization (feelings of being detached from oneself);
- fear of losing control or going crazy;
- fear of dying;
- numbing or tingling sensations;
- chills or hot flushes.

Thus people who have panic attacks have a combination of these symptoms. Many have not just four, but five, six, seven or even all 13! People with PTSD are very prone to panic attacks, which may be triggered by memories of the traumatic event. However, they often come out of the blue. Although people may feel an overwhelming sense of dread when in panic, they are often reassured when told that these symptoms are harmless and caused by the body experiencing a huge surge of arousal in response to stress. However, in many cases of PTSD, panic attacks develop into a pattern that causes significant distress, with a resultant reduction in quality of life.

There are some simple rules for managing a panic attack.

- Remember that panic attacks will subside naturally over minutes rather than hours (panic is a state of extreme 'fight or flight', and the body can only maintain the highest levels of physical arousal for relatively short periods).
- Panic attacks do not lead to death or heart attacks – therefore try to stay calm. Think to yourself: 'This is a panic attack – the feeling will pass.'
- Sit or lie down if you can – try not to rush around, which will increase the feelings.
- Try to slow your breathing and to breathe from the diaphragm. During panic attacks, overbreathing – sometimes called hyperventilation (see below) – makes the symptoms worse because it causes the loss of too much carbon dioxide from the body.
- The old remedy of re-breathing expired air from a paper bag is effective within minutes. This method simply puts back carbon dioxide into the body and restores the correct balance of blood gases. Remember that even extreme hyperventilation will cause no real harm.
- Avoid taking tranquillizing medication or alcohol. The panic will probably pass before these substances have time to act.

Hyperventilation

Hyperventilation (overbreathing) occurs in states of high anxiety. This is one of the body's mechanisms for dealing with 'fight or flight', by taking in as much oxygen as possible to feed your muscles for activity. The problem with the hyperventilation of anxiety is that there is no fight or flight to deal with, and you breathe out carbon dioxide too quickly. This leads to a change in the acidity of the body (which is harmless). However, this change in body acidity leads to a number of symptoms, such as pins and needles, light-headedness, chest pain or discomfort – indeed many of the symptoms described above.

Hyperventilation can occur in several different ways:

1 There may be an increased breathing rate – as I have said above, breathing quickens in a state of fight or flight. Sometimes this is obvious, but often breathing quickens in its rate slowly and imperceptibly, over a period of time. The net result is the same – a change in the acidity of the body.
2 Some people have a tendency to take unnecessary deep breaths when they become anxious; often such individuals have a tendency to yawn. One of the main issues with hyperventilation is that your body starts to feel shortness of breath. It feels as though it's not getting enough oxygen and you breathe unnecessarily deeply, when the problem is actually the opposite.
3 The more you think about breathing, the more you breathe – thus you begin to hyperventilate!

In Chapter 11 there is specific advice about relaxation and breathing exercises and meditation, as techniques for managing anxiety, with information about useful resources.

9

Coping with anger, guilt and depression

Anger and irritability are very common problems in PTSD, because the body has been put into a state of heightened 'fight or flight' and, simply put, one's fuse is much shorter. Sometimes anger and irritability come out of the blue but more often than not, if you keep a record of these episodes, you will find that there is a pattern associated with many of the outbursts, linked to particular triggers. Thus keeping a diary is very important, noting what situation you were in at the time the problem arose and what may have been going through your mind. Many people are helped by the revelation that particular situations cause angry outbursts. As we have noted elsewhere in the book, anger is an emotion that may be wrapped up with guilty feelings – thus, in the case of a parent who has lost a child, seeing happy parents and their children on the street will evoke angry thoughts and feelings, such as 'Why are they happy and I am not?', 'Why have they got a healthy child and my child died?' or 'I feel so angry about the doctor who gave me the wrong advice.'

In such cases there is often guilt – for example, guilt for feeling that other people do not deserve healthy children or, in the case of the negligent doctor, guilt that one also had a responsibility for detecting medical problems. Anticipating a trigger will, in itself, be helpful in preventing the anger arising. One very common and effective method of dealing with anger is to reduce physical arousal. Arousal reduction can be much assisted by the use of exercise, relaxation, breathing techniques or mindfulness. These useful, practical, approaches – used alone or in combination – are to be strongly recommended for dealing with angry thoughts. I must emphasize that mindfulness, relaxation and breathing exercises all need to be practised regularly, and that it may be some time before significant benefit accrues. Similarly with exercise: one run may serve to diffuse angry feelings for the moment, but it is only over a period of time, with practice of regular exercise, that the long-term beneficial effects will be felt.

Although avoidance in PTSD can, in general, be problematic, there may be a need simply to take yourself out of situations that cause significant upset and anger until you have learned the relevant coping strategy.

Many people with problems associated with outbursts of anger or irritability will report that they have used alcohol to calm themselves down. Although alcohol sometimes works as a short-term remedy, in general those with any significant levels of anger or irritability should consider abstaining from it completely. It is well known that alcohol worsens problems associated with anger and irritability. Overall, one needs to remember that it is a central-nervous-system depressant, and that after a relatively short period of time, when the more euphoric effects of alcohol have worn off, the person will be left in a more subdued and irritable state and so be more vulnerable to angry outbursts. In the immediate period after consuming alcohol it of course leads to a feeling of relaxation, but this is often accompanied by disinhibition, and one may not foresee the consequences of one's actions. Disinhibition often leads to an increase in angry outbursts.

The American Psychological Association has a great website on controlling anger that gives some very useful advice – see <www.apa.org/topics/anger/control.aspx>.

Coping with guilt

Guilt can be an overwhelming problem for those with PTSD, as the following case history demonstrates.

The case of Susie

At the time of the accident Susie was a 31-year-old doctor, having just become a GP following several years of training. She had been visiting her parents in another city and was returning to her home, driving on a motorway. As Susie had had a lot of experience in her medical training of seeing people suffering the devastating results of road traffic accidents, she was, as usual, driving very carefully, making sure she left sufficient space between her car and the car in front and observing the speed limit at all times. The roads were quiet and Susie overtook in the correct manner, moving out and then back into the slower lane after indicating. While travelling at about 105 km/65 miles per hour, Susie pulled out to overtake a vehicle travelling in the middle lane. Suddenly this vehicle veered into her path and Susie braked immediately and attempted to take evasive action. Susie's car hit the central reservation barrier and spun several times, eventually skidding across the hard shoulder and rolling down an embankment – the car turning over at least three times. Susie remained conscious throughout and recalls the whole accident happening 'in slow motion'. She vividly recalls seeing smoke coming from the front of her car and thinking that she was going to be killed in an explosion. She was unable to release herself from her seatbelt and was trapped by a badly damaged door. She also recalls seeing 'blood everywhere'. Susie was rescued by emergency services following a prolonged attempt to release her from the wreckage. The feeling that she was about to die increased, and by the time she was put into the ambulance, she recalls shaking and crying inconsolably. On arrival at the hospital Susie was examined and, somewhat miraculously, she had no major injuries apart from a very bad cut on her forehead that was the cause of the bleeding. She was seen quickly, by the specialist plastic surgery team, who took her to the operating theatre and tended to the wound on her head. Susie was discharged from hospital after a couple of days but, unfortunately, she had facial scarring, which in the months to come remained quite significant. She underwent several surgical procedures to deal with the scarring but she was eventually left with a considerable level of disfigurement. Susie was referred to an NHS specialist, who in turn referred her to someone with expertise in camouflaging make-up, which helped her cope with resuming her professional life, where she needed to face patients every working day.

So where does the guilt come in?

Susie, understandably, had a significant level of shock following the accident. She developed flashbacks in the form of vivid 'slow motion' images of the accident and was woken at night by dreams of being trapped in her car. These dreams were followed by panic attacks.

Susie was referred to me about six weeks after the accident and, over the months, I was able to help her deal with some of the symptoms of PTSD. However, the most significant symptom she experienced was an overwhelming feeling of guilt. It transpired that the driver who had suddenly swerved into her path had been using a mobile phone, this distraction apparently being the cause of the accident. This driver was killed because the car she was driving turned over and was struck by a lorry in the slow lane. Despite reassurance from various individuals, including the police officer responsible for investigating the accident, Susie had an enormous sense of guilt that she was responsible for killing the other driver. Indeed even though on several subsequent occasions – including by the coroner at the inquest – Susie was told that she was not in any way to blame, Susie's feeling of responsibility continued. It was only after several attempts by me to help her see her responsibilities in a rational light that it became evident that alongside the guilt, Susie also felt great anger towards the other driver for causing her facial disfigurement. Thus the source of her distress appeared to be not only her guilt that in some way she might have caused the accident but also her guilt at feeling angry at the woman who had died. It took some time to help Susie resolve the conundrum, and what appeared to be effective was to help her see that her feelings of anger towards the other driver were understandable and reasonable. It was only after Susie had recognized that her guilt about feeling angry was underpinning the more general overarching feeling of guilt that the problems began to diminish. She then decided that what she needed to do was to try to 'forget' the other driver who, although her actions by using a mobile phone were irresponsible in the extreme, was – like all of us – a human being who could do something that could potentially harm others. Susie also recognized that the angry feelings she was experiencing towards the other driver were serving in a destructive way to worsen her own distress. She used diary-keeping to, in her own words, 'put the angry feelings out of my head on to paper'. At the end of each week she took her diary and ceremoniously burned it. In her mind she was symbolically burning her angry feelings.

I learned one lesson from Susie, namely that sometimes people work out for themselves a resolution of a particular problem, and that my job is simply to help people to help themselves. Susie continues to work as a GP. She also eventually resumed the activities and hobbies that she had previously enjoyed outside of her working life. She told me recently that her training as a doctor and as a GP was 'of no use whatsoever' when it came to overcoming her PTSD, and that although she had attended courses on PTSD, she needed professional help to deal with her symptoms because she felt 'powerless' over her feelings.

Coping with depression

While people with PTSD will inevitably have depressive symptoms, those who have suffered serious physical injuries with permanent consequences will usually experience additional depressive symptoms because of their lost health or because of mobility problems. Another source of depression may occur in those with such a level of PTSD that they are unable to work and become depressed because of the loss of income. In yet another case, those with PTSD who have such anger and irritability that they alienate others will become sad or depressed because of lost or severely damaged relationships. Some people with PTSD simply feel 'depressed', for not one but a very wide range of reasons.

What are the signs and symptoms of depression?

A cardinal symptom of depression is a prevailing feeling of sadness, which at times may be overwhelming. Those with depression often have guilty feelings, may be indecisive and may have disturbances of sleep or appetite. They are generally pessimistic about not only themselves but the world and the future in general. They often describe a lack of interest in others and physical feelings such as tiredness. They commonly complain of a lack of interest in sex. Severe states of depression often lead to weight loss – often of 10 kg/1.5 stones or more – and feelings of being physically unwell. Many people with depression may tell you that they lack motivation and give up interest in hobbies and activities that they used to enjoy. They may become extremely dissatisfied with their work, and their performance at work may suffer.

At this point it is worth noting that feelings of sadness, misery and depression may lead to thoughts that you might wish to harm yourself in some way. If these thoughts are frequent or such that you feel there is a real risk, you must discuss them with your doctor or therapist. On this topic, please be assured that telling your doctor or therapist about these thoughts will not lead to your being 'sectioned' and admitted to hospital; rather, disclosure will lead to your receiving the help you need. The old cliché, 'a problem shared is a problem halved', is certainly true when it comes to feelings of self-harm. Similarly, many people with PTSD have the thought that they would be better off dead. If you have such thoughts, you should discuss them with your GP or therapist.

What can you do to cope with feelings of depression?

As we have noted before, in the case of the more severe levels of depression, antidepressant medication may often be very useful. Sometimes specific psychological therapy to deal with feeling depressed, such as cognitive behavioural therapy, will help you by focusing on thoughts, beliefs, attitudes and behaviours. CBT is available on the NHS and is provided by therapists who have received appropriate education and training. There are also a number of self-help methods that may be as effective as receiving help from a therapist. Paul Gilbert's book *Overcoming Depression* is widely recommended through the NHS and by others (full details are in the Further reading section at the end of this book). There are also a number of online and CD programmes – also widely recommended in the NHS – increasingly used as self-help methods.

MoodGym

One of the longest-established online – and free – programmes is MoodGym, an interactive programme designed to deal with depression. This was developed at the Australian National University at Canberra. One of the main reasons for its development was the fact that a very large number of people in Australia don't have easy access to health professionals, therefore web-based programmes are particularly useful for those living in rural and remote areas. MoodGym now has around 750,000 registered users. After entering an email address and unique password, anything about users remains anonymous. Those responsible for the development of the programme made it clear from the outset – and continue to make it clear through the website – that MoodGym is not a substitute for seeking a diagnosis and treatment from a professional, but may be very helpful as a method of self-help. Indeed many clinicians – including myself – tell people that it is a site well worth a look and can be used as an adjunct to any professional therapy they receive. I also need to make it clear that while interactive web-based programmes such as MoodGym are, in general, well liked by those who use them, and there is substantial evidence of their effectiveness, not everyone likes this form of help – some people simply prefer to speak to another human being! Others dislike using the internet (for a wide range of reasons), and prefer more traditional self-help methods such as books, CDs and audiotapes. The MoodGym programme consists of five modules, an inter-active game, assessments of anxiety and depression, downloadable relaxation audio recordings, a workbook and feedback assessment. The whole programme is underpinned by the principles of cogni-tive behavioural therapy, aimed to demonstrate the relationship between thoughts and emotions and working through dealing with stress and relationship break-ups as well as teaching relaxation and meditation techniques. My advice here is simple: why not give it a try? See <www.moodgym.anu.edu.au>. If you don't like it, don't use it; if you do like it, give it time. You can bookmark the section where you log out and resume when you log on again. Many people use MoodGym for just a few minutes a day rather than spending lengthy periods at a time.

The Australian government has now launched another – also free – online programme for treating depression. To access this, log on to <www.mindhealthconnect.org.au>.

The number of internet resources continues to grow, including those focused on children and adolescents. One such, called Catch It – ID, is a programme developed in Chicago and Boston and aimed at adolescents. An excellent review of these programmes may be found at: <www.ncbi.nlm.nih.gov/pubmed/20528700>.

The NHS uses a programme called Beating the Blues that is also used in a number of other countries. It consists of eight 50-minute sessions that help you deal with a wide range of symptoms of depression and anxiety. The programme is available, via your GP, on the NHS, but at present patients cannot access it directly. The reason is that Beating the Blues is a commercial product, and the costs of development – which were considerable – are returned by charging the NHS. Enter 'self-help therapies' into the search box at the NHS Choices website – <www.nhs.uk> – and you will find a wide range of advice about resources available.

Behavioural activation

One of the most important treatment approaches, and certainly one that is as effective as traditional CBT, is behavioural activation. This is particularly important as a means of self-help because the treatment method is – compared with many psychological therapies – very straightforward and easy to understand. I recommend an excellent book on behavioural activation at the end of this section. The approach is also recommended by the National Institute for Health and Care Excellence (NICE) in their guideline for the treatment of depression.

Behavioural activation is a very important treatment approach for PTSD because apart from depressed mood, it focuses on other important aspects of PTSD, including poor levels of motivation, avoidance behaviour and loss of interest. More than 30 years ago an American psychologist, Charles Ferster, described a model of depression based on the principles of learning. Ferster simply observed that when people become depressed they use escape and avoidance of thoughts and feelings and various situations as a method of coping. Although in one sense this reduction in behaviour prevents people facing what they perceive as distressing, what also happens is that they begin to engage less with activities that give them pleasure and satisfaction. In psychological terms, they receive less reinforcement. Quite simply, Ferster and others developed treatment approaches along the lines of increasing the amount of pleasurable and everyday behaviour and reducing avoidance. These are the approaches now called behavioural activation.

In recent years a number of research studies have shown that not only can behavioural activation be as effective as CBT, but also as effective as antidepressant medication. Behavioural activation has been used as a treatment method for people with all levels of depression – from mild to the most severe. Indeed it is used in inpatient settings where people with the most severe levels of depression receive treatment.

If you are to use behavioural activation as a self-help approach, one of the most important issues is first to define your level of activity. This can be accomplished by keeping a diary of what you do from day to day. Alongside this exercise you should also keep a record of what you have avoided in each day and why you have avoided it. For example, you might have avoided going out to see a friend because you felt you could not cope or that you might let yourself down in some way and your friends would think badly of you. More specifically, you might record that you don't go out to meet a friend because you 'can't be bothered'. Thus keeping a diary of what you do and what you avoid is a really good starting point.

Once you have kept a diary for a few days, you might then list all the things that you used to take part in that you either avoid completely or do much less. Such items might include only using your football season ticket once in three games; avoiding the cinema; declining invitations to parties and functions; not going fishing; not going to a yoga class; not going line dancing; not going to a book club; not walking for pleasure or not inviting friends home. This way you have a good picture of the current situation and a good picture of what 'normal' life and activities might look like. When I conduct an assessment of a patient in professional therapy, I use discussion as one of my central methods – discussing with patients their likes and dislikes, and particularly identifying avoided behaviours. If you are using behavioural activation as a self-help method, you should share this section of the book with a family member or friend – someone who might work with you to put behavioural activation into action.

The next stage in behavioural activation is a process called activity scheduling. At its simplest, activity scheduling means increasing one's level of behaviour in a graduated way over a number of weeks and trying, one by one, to engage in behaviours you have either avoided or have reduced in frequency. One of the most important principles here is to list these avoided behaviours in a hierarchical form; that is, with those that are most difficult to achieve at the top and those easier to achieve at the bottom of the list. One should then try to tackle behaviours from the bottom of the list and, in increasing doses of difficulty over days and weeks, work your way up the hierarchy.

In my experience it is very important to pace yourself realistically. Do not try to do too much too soon, but use the principle of doing things not only in a graduated way but tackling tasks that are *difficult but manageable*. Trying to do too much too soon may lead to the worsening of a sense of failure and thoughts such as, 'I knew I could never overcome this problem'. If you have a family member or friend who can assist you, he or she may be able to help you judge the speed at which you increase your level of activity and support and encourage you through setbacks. Indeed in my experience it is extremely unusual to complete a course of behavioural activation without experiencing one or more setbacks.

Continuing to keep a diary is very important in monitoring progress. It is always helpful to look back over the past days and weeks to reflect on how much progress has been made. It is also important to see how your thinking has changed and whether your predictions have been realized – for example, that going out with a friend will lead to a number of negative consequences. What usually happens is that you find that exposing yourself to situations that you have avoided will help you disconfirm your expectations and thus disconfirm your worst fears.

If you are to embark on a programme of behavioural activation without the assistance of a therapist, I recommend that you use *Manage Your Mood* by David Veale and Rob Willson, which will serve as a very helpful resource (full details in the Further reading section at the end of this book).

10

Relationships

Dealing with the effects of PTSD on others

If you have PTSD, while reading this book you may have reflected on the effects of your condition on others. You may have thought about your angry outbursts, how you may have responded disproportionately to some trivial comment by a family member. Alternatively, you may have thought about the times you refused invitations to eat with friends, go to the cinema or see a football match. Sometimes people with PTSD are all too aware of its effect on others. However, sometimes – because of the nature of their particular form of PTSD – all their thinking tends to be inwardly directed and they do not realize just how much their condition affects other people.

Obviously it is very important to open up to others and talk about not just the triggering event but also to let those close to you know about your symptoms. In my experience the education of significant others is a very important step in helping people with PTSD rebuild their lives. Thus although those with PTSD need to focus on coping with symptoms, it is also important that they recognize the need to tell those closest to them about the problem, particularly how the PTSD may have caused behaviours that have a negative effect on others, such as outbursts of temper or withdrawal from normal interactions. By communicating in this way, they may then be able to begin to restore positive relationships and deal with the negative consequences of the PTSD on family and friends. They need to pick up the telephone, email or even write a letter! Reading this book is the obvious way for other people to obtain information to begin a process of recovery and repair. However, some people with PTSD will need to recognize that they have gone past the point where it is possible to restore previous close or friendly relationships. Sometimes their behaviour may be such that even when recovery takes place, there is nothing one can do to deal with, for example, the effects of angry outbursts or destructive or antisocial behaviour. Accepting the reality that a relationship is over – something I have seen several times in the case of people whose marriages have broken down – is far from easy. Nevertheless, in my experience some people with PTSD need to realize that part of the recovery process may involve – quite simply – building a new life.

Hopefully, the above comments will only apply to a small proportion of people with PTSD, and I thought long and hard whether or not to mention such a sensitive issue. However, I concluded that there will be people with PTSD whose behaviour is such that relationships have broken down, and I would not be doing justice to them to leave this topic out of the book. I also thought that addressing it might demonstrate just how serious a problem PTSD is and how it has such wide-ranging effects.

Reassurance seeking

Many people with PTSD will develop the habit of reassurance seeking. This perhaps reflects that they are in an extremely vulnerable state and seek out others to provide comfort and a feeling of safety. The continual seeking of reassurance may then follow and someone with PTSD may seek reassurance about a wide range of matters – everything from questions such as, 'Will I be all right?' before embarking on a journey to, 'I'm not going mad, am I?' While all human beings require some reassurance at some time in their lives, excessive reassurance seeking can become a problem in its own right, leading to such dependency on others that one loses all sense of autonomy and independence of thinking and behaviour. Sometimes reassurance seeking is confined to a particular family member or friend and, when interviewed, these individuals will tell you that the same question is asked over and over again in a manner that can only be described as obsessive.

How, then, do you cope with reassurance seeking?

First, it is important to recognize that reassurance seeking comes from vulnerability and is a genuine attempt to confirm that one is 'safe'. On the other hand, the seeking of reassurance can become meaningless – particularly when the same question is asked over and over again. My particular way of dealing with this problem is to bring together the person who asks for reassurance and the person to whom the questions are directed, and discuss the usefulness – or otherwise – of the reassurance-seeking habit. Very quickly one comes to establish that reassurance seeking is indeed meaningless, and moreover that it can replace other, healthy conversations and interactions. I then ask the reassurance seeker and the person involved in giving reassurance to put a ban on the habit. At first this may cause anxiety because the person asking for reassurance will experience some short-term relief, albeit this is replaced in minutes or seconds by the need for yet more reassurance! All habits, including reassurance seeking, may be difficult to break, but in my experience a total ban on the habit is the most effective way of dealing with the problem.

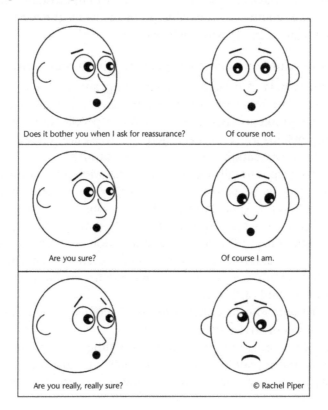

Coping with sexual difficulties

Sexual difficulties are an extremely common manifestation of trauma in people who have been involved in various accidents, who are the victims of robberies or who have suffered war-related events.

The emotional numbing that occurs in PTSD is often a feature of these sexual difficulties. People with PTSD very often feel that they are unable to connect intimately with their partners. In some cases, even when sexual activity is attempted, various problems then arise. Men may, for example, be unable to obtain an erection or may experience premature ejaculation. Women often complain of pain during intercourse or are unable to reach sexual orgasm. In most cases, PTSD patients will tell me that their interest in sex is either much diminished or absent.

Those who have been sexually assaulted will in most, but not all, cases also encounter considerable problems when they attempt to resume sexual activity with their partner.

How then does one begin to deal with sexual problems?

Sometimes it is important to obtain help and to see a suitably trained professional with expertise in the assessment and treatment of sexual problems. However, sometimes people can overcome sexual problems using self-help methods. These are certainly worth trying before embarking on professional treatment.

The first step is to talk about the problem with your partner. This is essential because partners often feel they have been 'shut out' and have had no explanation about the reasons why sexual activity has either been reduced or become absent. Simply educating your partner about how PTSD leads to a diminution or absence of sexual function is reassuring, and they should therefore benefit from reading this book (see also my recommendations concerning other books at the end of this section).

While there is no easy answer to sexual problems, there are some useful pieces of advice that may assist.

One of the most important things in telling your partner of the difficulty and explaining that you are unable to take part in sexual activity in the way you used to, is to say very clearly that this does not mean you do not love him or her. Furthermore, it is also often helpful to tell your partner that you are frustrated at not being able to show that you do love and care.

You should try to ensure that you have as much physical contact as possible – hold hands, put your arms around each other and generally 'cuddle up' as much as possible. However, in the early stages it is important that you and your partner come to an agreement that you will not take part in any sexual activity whatsoever until you are both comfortable with non-sexual touching.

You also need to ensure that you spend time together and do things that might relax your mood – for example, going for a walk, having a meal out, going to the cinema or, very simply, sitting down together and watching a favourite TV programme or listening to music. Sometimes these activities are best carried out when you have tried to relax by using a relaxation, breathing or meditation exercise (see Chapter 11).

As you progress, you might then be able to move things on by giving each other a gentle, non-sexual massage using oils or lotions, rubbing the back of each other's neck or shoulders. You should ensure that you spend an equal amount of time giving the other person pleasure. Ask your partner what he or she enjoys – some people like their legs to be massaged, or their feet, others just simply enjoy a shoulder rub.

You might then, when you feel comfortable doing so, progress from this stage to more sexually orientated activities, but without full intercourse. This graduated approach to dealing with sexual problems forms the basis of most sex-therapy programmes delivered by professionals.

Two books that I know have been helpful to many couples and that are often recommended by other professionals are Vicki Ford's *Overcoming Sexual Problems* and Helen Kennerley's *Overcoming Childhood Trauma* (full details are in the Further reading section at the end of this book).

11

Mindfulness, relaxation and exercise

In this chapter I will describe in more detail the use of three particular approaches I have mentioned in previous chapters and that are often very helpful in dealing with a number of the problems associated with PTSD. However, it is worth emphasizing that these do not in any way replace the central treatments for PTSD that I discussed in Chapter 4: trauma-focused cognitive behavioural therapy (CBT) or eye movement desensitization and reprocessing (EMDR), used alone or in combination with one of the medications recommended by the National Institute for Health and Care Excellence (NICE).

Mindfulness

Mindfulness is now used widely in the NHS as a treatment, particularly for depression. However, in my opinion it may be a very useful approach for those with PTSD. It may be particularly useful for dealing with distressing intrusive memories or at times when you become preoccupied by particular thoughts and feelings.

To begin, I have to say that mindfulness is not a new therapy developed by psychologists; it is in fact an approach based on Buddhist practice, of which mindfulness is deemed a central part. A generally accepted definition of mindfulness reads as follows:

> The intentional accepting and non judgmental focusing of one's attention on the emotions, thoughts and sensations of being in the present moment.

Mindfulness is therefore a method of meditating and has been developed as a range of techniques used in mental health practice in the past 35 years or so. The Mental Health Foundation, a leading UK charity, has a downloadable podcast on its website for a ten-minute practice exercise – see <www.mentalhealth.org.uk/help-

information/podcasts/mindfulness-10-minute/?view=Standard>. This very helpful exercise is narrated by Professor Mark Williams, one of the UK's leading psychologists and someone who has researched the effectiveness of mindfulness in a number of research programmes. The exercise lasts about ten minutes. In my experience, it is useful as a method of dealing with the upsurge of particular emotions, such as anxiety and anger, and can also be helpful for people who experience intrusive memories and flashbacks. The Mental Health Foundation offers a great deal of information about the availability of mindfulness. In my opinion, attending a mindfulness course is often helpful, particularly as it brings together individuals seeking solutions to various problems connected with anxiety and depression. Having said that, I also know of many people who have been able to acquire mindfulness skills through self-help books – for example, Shamash Alidina's *Mindfulness for Dummies* (full details are in the Further reading section at the end of this book).

Relaxation

Relaxation techniques may be helpful in reducing the general level of physical arousal and body tension. The instructions that follow will provide advice on how to employ the technique. Otherwise, there are various relaxation exercises available on CDs or in other forms.

While there are many ways to achieve relaxation, most focus on a systematic tensing and relaxing of the muscles in the body. This has two benefits. First, it helps you differentiate between states of tension and relaxation and, importantly, recognize when your level of muscle tension is increasing. Second, there is considerable evidence to suggest that systematic tensing and relaxing exercises eventually lead to a state of overall muscle relaxation and as a consequence a feeling of well-being.

The following instructions are straightforward. It may be helpful to read and inwardly digest them, then make a recording that you can follow. If you do this, however, remember to leave a 10-second gap between each phase. This may be as effective as any commercially available recording and is certainly worth trying, as unlike them it is free!

First of all, identify a time in the day when you have 30 minutes to devote to this task. Find a quiet room, turn off your mobile, unplug the landline and wear loose, comfortable clothing. The exercise can be carried out in a comfortable chair or lying down, and you should experiment with different situations and times of the day to identify what the optimum conditions are for you.

Before doing the exercises it is important to remember that, when tensing your muscles, this should be done to a moderate extent. If you tense them too hard you will defeat the object of the exercise. A simple guide is that it should lead to no more than a sensation of tensing or 'pulling'. If you experience pain you are trying too hard. Further, when you release the tension, you should feel it go immediately.

Get in position and begin with your right hand. Clench your fist so that your knuckles are white. Hold for 5 seconds, then release immediately.

Pause, wait 10 seconds, then repeat.

Tense your right forearm, closing your fist and tensing the muscles of your forearm. Remember: not too hard. Hold for 5 seconds, then release immediately.

Pause, wait 10 seconds, then repeat.

Tense your right biceps, clenching your fist and bending your arm, so that it forms a 90° angle. Concentrate on making your biceps bulge as much as possible. Hold for 5 seconds, then release immediately.

Pause, wait 10 seconds, then repeat.

Repeat these actions with the left hand, forearm and biceps. Remembering to do each exercise twice, hold for 5 seconds, then release immediately.

Next move your head and neck. Tense your eye muscles. Screw up your eyes and keep them shut tight. Hold for 5 seconds, then release immediately.

Pause, wait 10 seconds, then repeat.

Tense your mouth by clenching your jaws together and concentrate on pressing your lips together as firmly as possible. At the same time, you will notice that you tense your eyes. Hold for 5 seconds, then release immediately.

Pause, wait 10 seconds, then repeat.

Now concentrate on tensing your neck. Push your chin down a little towards your chest but do not touch your chest. Hold for 5 seconds, then release immediately.

Pause, wait 10 seconds, then repeat.

Next, move your shoulders and back, pushing your shoulders up slightly and tensing your neck. Feel the muscles tighten across your shoulders. Hold for 5 seconds, then release immediately.

Pause, wait 10 seconds, then repeat.

Tense your shoulders and arms by pushing your arms down, holding your neck rigid. Concentrate on tensing across your shoulders. Hold for 5 seconds, then release immediately.

Pause, wait 10 seconds, then repeat.

Tense the muscles in your back by pushing your elbows into your sides, pulling your shoulders down, holding your neck tight and pushing your head down towards your chest and concentrate on tensing the muscles across your back. Hold for 5 seconds, then release immediately.

Pause, wait 10 seconds, then repeat.

Now move to your chest and abdomen. Tense the muscles of your chest by pushing your shoulders back, pushing your elbows down into your waist and tilting your head back slightly and concentrate on holding your chest in a barrel-like, rigid way. Hold for 5 seconds, then release immediately.

Pause, wait 10 seconds, then repeat.

Tense the muscles of your stomach from the back and pull in towards your navel. Hold for 5 seconds, then release immediately.

Pause, wait 10 seconds, then repeat.

Next, move to your lower body and legs. Tense your thighs and buttocks by pushing your buttocks down and concentrate on tensing your thighs and buttocks together. Hold for 5 seconds, then release immediately.

Pause, wait 10 seconds, then repeat.

Tense your right calf by pulling your toes up towards you, keeping your leg straight at the knee. Pull your toes back until you can feel the pull all the way up your calf muscles. Hold for 5 seconds, then release immediately.

Pause, wait 10 seconds, then repeat.

Tense your right foot by curling over your toes, trying to make your toes clench like a fist. Hold for 5 seconds, then release immediately.

Pause, wait 10 seconds, then repeat.

Repeat this sequence for your left calf and foot.

When you come to this point, begin to tense your whole body, starting with your hands, working up through your arms, then head, neck, shoulders, back, chest, stomach, buttocks, thighs, calves and feet. Take 10 seconds to gradually tense the whole body. Hold for 5 seconds, then relax.

As you relax, breathe out as much as you can, slowly. Keep your eyes closed and say 'calm' to yourself.

Repeat this sequence 5 times, remembering to leave 10 seconds between each.

Next, concentrate on slowing down your breathing. Try to feel all your chest and, as you breath out, say 'calm' to yourself. Let your breathing settle into a natural rhythm and then try to fix your mind on a quiet and relaxing scene. Imagine yourself lying on a beach or in a meadow. Imagine a warm atmosphere around you. Try to image the smells of this environment. Keep your mind as fixed on this place as possible and let yourself drift. Don't worry if you fall asleep, but perhaps it may be worth setting your alarm clock first!

Breathing exercises

Breathing exercises are probably one of the most effective ways of dealing with high levels of anxiety and they are also helpful at times when you simply need to calm down. Controlling your breathing not only gives you a feeling of calm but also reduces your blood pressure and generally reduces stress on the body. Remember that breathing should involve all the chest and diaphragm. Breathing from the top of the chest – the anxious breathing that we all experience at times – promotes more anxiety.

Simple breathing exercises

One of the most important things about controlled breathing is to slow down your breathing rate gradually, so that eventually you are breathing 6–8 times a minute, instead of 14, 16 or more. Simply find somewhere to relax (a nice comfortable chair is better than a bed), put one hand at the top of your chest and the other on your upper abdomen. Breathe in through your nose, making sure the whole chest inflates. You can feel this by the movement in your hands. Breathe very slowly in. Hold it and then exhale slowly.

Another trick that is often used is alternate-nostril breathing, something often practised in yoga classes. Sit for a while in a comfortable chair and relax as much as possible. Then place your right thumb over your right nostril and breathe in through your left nostril. When you have taken in a deep breath, close off your left nostril and exhale through your right nostril. Continue this breathing for 5–10 minutes – it really works. Breathing exercises often work well after you have practised deep-muscle relaxation techniques.

As I noted in Chapter 7, I often recommend a 'quick fix' breathing exercise available on a podcast of the Mental Health Foundation – again, see <www.mentalhealth.org.uk/help-information/podcasts/ stress-relaxation-quick-fix/>.

Many people advocate using a breathing or relaxation technique twice a day. Although this may take up 45 minutes or so, you will find that for the rest of the day you feel much calmer, and actually your efficiency in everyday tasks will be increased if you are more relaxed.

Physical exercise

We all need physical exercise and there is considerable evidence that it is essential for keeping in good health. On the other hand, there is also plentiful evidence that exercise levels are declining and that a lack of exercise is linked with a greatly increased risk of developing a number of health problems, notably those affecting the heart and circulation and also connected with the weight problems that affect many people who do not exercise. Having said that, it is clear that people of normal weight who do not exercise are also very prone to developing a number of physical illnesses.

For people with PTSD, exercise is particularly important. There is now considerable evidence that participating in jogging, yoga and strength training leads to a reduction in anxiety levels and improvement in mood. Research studies show that people who participate in exercise programmes show improved self-esteem, better levels of social interaction and, importantly, a reduction in symptoms of depression, as I shall discuss in a moment. Research has also found that exercise participants showed an increase in motivation, which in turn leads to paying more attention to healthy eating and hygiene.

With regard to those with PTSD who have mild to moderate depression, NICE recommends exercise as a first-line treatment, and a number of studies show that, for this condition, exercise can be as beneficial as antidepressants or talking therapies.

For people with PTSD who are taking medications, exercise is also important because the medications used may have a tendency to promote weight gain. Weight gain itself leads to an inactive lifestyle, and so a vicious circle develops.

Which type of exercise is beneficial?

The answer to this is anything that gets you active, and simple exercise, such as walking instead of driving or being conveyed as a passenger, gardening, playing with children are all beneficial. However, just keeping an active lifestyle by walking or gardening is, in all probability, not enough. It is important that we exercise to the level that we – simply put – get our heart and lungs going, and so reasonable exercise will involve getting breathless. One simple rule of thumb is that beneficial exercise should involve getting out of breath, but not so much that you can't say a few words, sing a little or hold a simple conversation. For many, simply brisk walking will get them out of breath, but for most people it is necessary to jog, cycle, swim or go to the gym.

How do you start an exercise programme?

As people with PTSD may have difficulty getting started because of either avoidance behaviours or poor levels of motivation (or both), family members or carers can assist by engaging in the exercise regime with them. This may mean putting aside half an hour to go for a jog or a swim or signing up together at the gym. Your GP may be able to organize exercise on prescription, starting you off with a number of free supervised sessions at a local leisure centre.

Exercise on prescription

If you want to know about exercise on prescription, go to the website NHS Choices – <www.nhs.uk> – and type in 'exercise'. You will probably find that the first page that comes up concerns exercise for depression. This is because depression is one of the commonest conditions for which GPs can prescribe exercise. However, people with significant levels of PTSD are entitled to exercise on prescription. The website will tell you that adults should be active for at least 150 minutes (2 hours and 30 minutes) each week. However, there is plentiful evidence that most adults of working age require more than this to obtain maximum benefits. One of the great advantages of exercise on prescription is that it will get you started. If you have done nothing for several years, you will not be able to exercise at reasonable levels for 150 minutes a week. You will probably need to start with a few minutes and build up.

Note: Should you have any health problems, take any regular medication, or should you have been inactive for a lengthy period, you should consult your GP before embarking on a programme of exercise.

Finally, taking exercise may have more general benefits. Joining a cycling or running club, a zumba class or keep-fit session will bring the benefits of social interaction. The vast majority of these activities make no stipulation about ability and indeed most running clubs, for example, will encourage absolute beginners to join and offer coaching aimed at simply getting one started. Apart from events such as the Race for Life runs and walks organized by Cancer Research UK that are held all over the UK (<http://raceforlife.cancerresearchuk.org/index.html>), there are now Park Runs held in nearly 300 locations (<www.parkrun.org.uk>). These events are held in local parks, are free to enter, happen every Saturday at 9 a.m. and involve a 5 km (3 mile) run/walk.

Conclusion

Writing this book has been a revelation for me in many ways. Although my experience of assessing and treating people with PTSD extends over more than 35 years and includes seeing people suffering from the widest range of traumatic events, and although research has revealed much, I can see that there is still a great deal to be learned. There is so much that we don't know. Part of the incomplete knowledge of the condition and its treatment relates to the way individuals respond after trauma. As I have shown in some of the case histories here, people react in their own individual ways, and some recover from PTSD without any particular treatment. When one tries to find out why they have recovered, often no obvious answers are apparent. I think I have concluded that professional treatment can offer a great deal but rarely provides the complete answer. On reflecting on the stories of several of the people I have seen, I have also learned that some of the most traumatized and vulnerable individuals are also in their own way resilient; they may continue to be productive members of society and sometimes, despite their suffering, can demonstrate a great sense of humour.

What has this book conveyed?

First, I suppose, that PTSD is a new term describing a condition that has probably always been a feature of human existence. Second, PTSD is much more common than one would imagine, and the various forms can present with a wide range of signs and symptoms that can affect the most basic activities of daily living. PTSD does not always need professional treatment – some people simply improve with time. With regard to complex cases, I think that what has been learned is that in cases of physical injury, the psychological and the physical become intertwined and one should never separate completely the treatment approaches. Sadly, because of the way that health services operate, it is almost as if those responsible for delivering psychological therapies are oblivious to those attempting treatment and rehabilitation for physical injuries and vice versa. At the present time it is rare that those with complex physical problems, as well as PTSD, receive a thoroughly integrated treatment approach, with care co-ordination.

A main aim of this book has been to provide, as in Part 2, a number of ways of coping with the many manifestations of PTSD. No doubt there are problems I have not described and, for some of the problem areas, the advice I have provided has been somewhat limited. Nevertheless, my hope is that this book will be read and then kept as a resource and that it may offer practical assistance for those with PTSD and those close to them. Finally, let me turn once more to the person to whom this book is dedicated, my own father, Joe. War certainly traumatized him. The scars from the machine-gun bullet wounds that led to his being in hospital for two years were plain to see on the day he died, aged 93. The psychological trauma was evident in the anxiety and vulnerability he showed to the family, although not to the outside world. However, he also demonstrated that the effects of trauma need not prevent one from leading a productive life. With hindsight, I can see that Joe developed his own ways of coping.

Useful addresses

PTSD and anxiety

Anxiety UK
Zion Community Resource Centre
339 Stretford Road
Hulme
Manchester M15 4ZY
Helpline: 08444 775 774 (Monday to Friday, 9.30 a.m. to 5.30 p.m.)
General enquiries: 0161 226 7727
Website: www.anxietyuk.org.uk

Assist Trauma Care
11 Albert Street
Rugby CV21 2RX
Tel.: 01788 551919
Website: www.assisttraumacare.org.uk

British Association for Behavioural and Cognitive Psychotherapies (BABCP)
Imperial House
Hornby Street
Bury BL9 5BN
Tel.: 0161 705 4304
Website: www.babcp.com

Combat Stress (Ex-Services Mental Welfare Society)
Tyrwhitt House
Oaklawn Road
Leatherhead
Surrey KT22 0BX
Helpline: 0800 138 1619
General enquiries: 01372 587 000
Website: www.combatstress.org.uk

Health and Care Professions Council
Park House
184 Kennington Park Road
London SE11 4BU
Tel.: 0845 300 6184
Website: www.hcpc-uk.org.uk

Mind
15–19 Broadway
Stratford
London E15 4BQ
Tel.: 020 8519 2122
Website: www.mind.org.uk

Mind Cymru
3rd Floor
Quebec House
Castlebridge
5–19 Cowbridge Road East
Cardiff CF11 9AB
Tel.: 029 2039 5123
Website: www.mind.org.uk

No Panic
Jubilee House
74 High Street
Madeley
Telford
Shropshire TF7 5AH
Helpline: 0844 967 4848 (every day, 10 a.m. to 10 p.m.)
Crisis number: 01952 680835 (a recorded message, available 24 hours
a day)
General enquiries: 01952 680 460
Website: www.nopanic.org.uk

The Northern Ireland Association for Mental Health
80 University Street
Belfast BT7 1HE
Tel.: 028 9032 8474
Website: www.niamhwellbeing.org

The Scottish Association for Mental Health
Brunswick House
51 Wilson Street
Glasgow G1 1UZ
Tel.: 0141 530 1000
Website: www.samh.org.uk

Victim Support
See website for addresses of local offices.
Supportline: 0845 30 30 900 (Monday to Friday, 8 a.m. to 8 p.m.;
weekends, 9 a.m. to 7 p.m.; bank holidays, 9 a.m. to 5 p.m.)
Website: www.victimsupport.org.uk

Other

Addaction
Tel.: 020 7251 5860
Website: www.addaction.org.uk

Alcoholics Anonymous (AA)
Tel.: 0800 769 7555
Website: www.alcoholics-anonymous.org.uk

Mental Health Foundation
Tel.: 020 7803 110
Website: www.mentalhealth.org.uk

National Health Service (NHS)
Website: www.nhs.uk

National Institute for Health and Care Excellence (NICE)
Tel. 0300 323 0140
Website: www.nice.org.uk

National Society for the Prevention of Cruelty to Children (NSPCC)
Free helpline: 0800 800 5000 (24 hours a day, 365 days a year)
Website: www.nspcc.org.uk

Samaritans
Website: www.samaritans.org

SANDS
Website: www.uk-sands.org

The Compassionate Friends
Website: www.tcf.org.uk

References

Beck, Judith (no date), 'What Is Cognitive Behavior Therapy?', <www.beck institute.org/cognitive-behavioral-therapy>.

Bentley, Steve (2005), 'A Short History of PTSD: From Thermopylae to Hue, soldiers have always had a disturbing reaction to war', *The VVA Veteran* March/April 2005, 27–30. (According to the magazine the article was originally published in 1991.)

Bisson, J. and Andrew, M. (2007), 'Psychological Treatment of Post-Traumatic Stress Disorder', *Cochrane Database of Systematic Reviews* (3), CD 003388.

Daly, R. J. (1983), 'Samuel Pepys and Post-Traumatic Stress Disorder', *British Journal of Psychiatry* 143(1), 64–8.

Gournay, Kevin (ed.) (1989), *Agoraphobia: Current perspectives on theory and treatment* (London: Routledge).

Locke, John (1693), *Some Thoughts Concerning Education* (London). This work is readily available to buy in modern reprints, including e-books, or to read cost-free online – for example at < www.bartleby.com/37/1>.

Shapiro, F. (1989), 'Efficacy of the Eye Movement Desensitization Procedure in the Treatment of Traumatic Memories', *Journal of Traumatic Stress* 2(2), 199–223.

Sherin, Jonathan E. and Nemeroff, Charles B. (2011), 'Post-Traumatic Stress Disorder: The neurobiological impact of psychological trauma', *Dialogues in Clinical Neuroscience* 13(3), 263–78 – available to read at <www.ncbi.nlm.nih.gov/pmc/articles/PMC3182008/>.

Further reading

Alidina, Shamash (2014), *Mindfulness for Dummies*, 2nd edn (London: Wiley).

Barker, Pat (1996), *The Regeneration Trilogy* (London: Viking).

Ford, Vicki, V. (2010), *Overcoming Sexual Problems: A self-help guide using cognitive behavioral techniques* (London: Constable & Robinson).

Gilbert, Paul (2009), *Overcoming Depression: A self-help guide using cognitive behavioral techniques*, 3rd edn (London: Constable & Robinson).

Johnston, Fiona (2000), *Getting a Good Night's Sleep: A handbook for people who have trouble sleeping* (London: Sheldon Press).

Kennerley, Helen H. (2009), *Overcoming Childhood Trauma: A self-help guide using cognitive behavioral techniques* (London: Constable & Robinson).

NICE (2005), *Post-Traumatic Stress Disorder (PTSD): The treatment of PTSD in adults and children. Understanding NICE guidance – information for people with PTSD, their advocates and carers, and the public* (London: NICE).

NICE (2005), *Post-Traumatic Stress Disorder: the management of PTSD in adults and children in primary and secondary care* (London: NICE).

Veale, David and Willson, Rob (2007), *Manage Your Mood: How to use behavioral activation techniques to overcome depression* (London: Constable & Robinson).

Index